CAREERS
IN ANESTHESIOLOGY

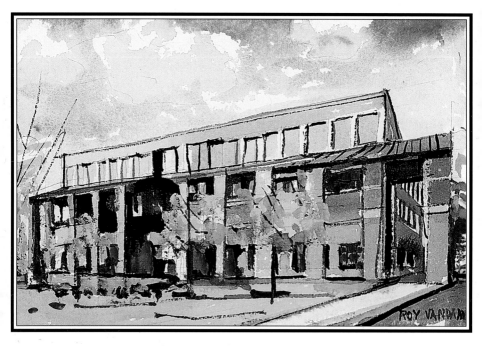

*Headquarters Building of the American Society of Anesthesiologists.
Almost one third of the three spacious floors is devoted to the
collections of the Wood Library-Museum.
(From a painting by Professor Leroy Vandam)*

CAREERS
IN ANESTHESIOLOGY

Autobiographical Memoirs

WILLIAM HAMILTON
No Time at All

ELI BROWN
An Autobiographical Essay

E.M. PAPPER
The Palate of My Mind

Edited by B. Raymond Fink

VOLUME I

THE
WOOD LIBRARY-MUSEUM
OF ANESTHESIOLOGY
PARK RIDGE, ILLINOIS
1997

Published By
Wood Library-Museum of Anesthesiology

Library of Congress Number 97-60921

Hard Cover Edition: ISBN 0-9614932-8-3
Paperback Edition: ISBN 0-9614932-9-1

Printed in the United States of America

Published by:
WOOD LIBRARY-MUSEUM
OF ANESTHESIOLOGY
520 N. Northwest Highway
Park Ridge, Illinois 60068-2573
(847) 825-5586 / FAX 847-825-1692
WLM@ASAhq.org

TABLE OF CONTENTS

WILLIAM HAMILTON
No Time at All
Page 1

ELI BROWN
An Autobiographical Essay
Page 41

E.M. PAPPER
The Palate of My Mind
Page 67

PUBLICATIONS COMMITTEE

B. Raymond Fink (Co-Chair)
C. Ronald Stephen (Co-Chair)
Doris K. Cope
Norig Ellison
Nicholas M. Greene
Kathryn E. McGoldrick
Susan A. Vassallo

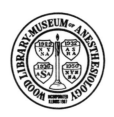

EDITOR'S NOTE

These memoirs inaugurate a new experiment in living history from the Wood Library-Museum of Anesthesiology. They present autobiographical panoramas of the protracted revolution which overtook anesthetic practice in the second half of the twentieth century. Principal participants here retell the motivations, actions, incidents and dominant events of their careers, virtually unburdened by limits of self-expression.

This volume pulsates with creative diversity, the throb of artisans busily weaving individual threads of their own making, into a tapestry more than a little reminiscent of a philosophy articulated by Chief Seattle at about the dawn of anesthesia.

This we know.

> *All things are connected*
> *like the blood*
> *which unites one family*

>> *Whatever befalls the earth*
>> *befalls the sons and daughters of the earth*

>>> *Man did not weave the web of life,*
>>> *he is merely a strand in it.*

>>>> *Whatever he does to the web*
>>>> *he does to himself.*

Someone has said that the unexamined life is not worth living. Well, here is a clutch of lives examined, found pre-eminently worth living—and most decidedly worth reading! As already indicated, they are distinguished invited cameos from the renascence of anesthesiology in World War II and its aftermath. Their sequence is fortuitously geographic, rotating with the planet from west to east. Others awaiting the next turn of the press are delayed only by the incompressibility of time.

For the present group of bedside pleasures, you and I are deeply indebted to WLM's Board of Trustees and Publications Committee, to prince of librarians Patrick Sim, to Sally Graham, stellar assistant librarian, to our production expert, Roz Pape, and to devoted staff working at the headquarters of the American Society of Anesthesiologists. Thanks to the exceptional vision of our Society, a large part of that comely building is Paul Wood Library-Museum territory. Inside and out, the entire edifice exudes pride and dedication to the ageless ideals of the physicians who planned, own, and use it. Leroy Vandam's evocative painting, frontispiece to this and subsequent volumes, reflects the subtle unifying role of the Society in the careers you are about to savor.

—B. Raymond Fink

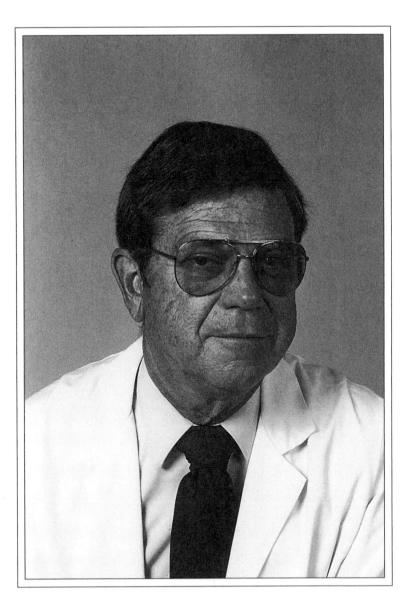

William Hamilton, M.D.

For Dennis
Bill Hamilton
ASA-1998

NO TIME
AT ALL

An
Autobiography

WILLIAM HAMILTON, M.D.

NO TIME AT ALL
An Autobiography

We are now observing the 150th anniversary of the birth of surgical anesthesia. It has been my destiny to participate in anesthesia for over one-third of that period, and it is of some interest to write a brief sketch of my professional career.

I first administered an anesthetic to a real patient in early March, 1946, a few months before the 100th anniversary of the first use of ether anesthesia in Boston on October 16, 1846. This event occurred near the end of my senior year in medical school. It happened because I was standing near the phone in the Division of Anesthesia at the University of Iowa College of Medicine. Dr. Stuart C. Cullen was the chief of that unit and personally answered the phone call which was a request from the Department of Otolaryngology to provide anesthesia to enable them to perform a myringotomy on a small child. Dr. Cullen asked me to accompany him. I doubt many department chairs are either answering service calls or taking medical students to answer such calls today.

We took a small bottle of Vinethene (divinyl ether), a small home-made gauze mask and, as I recall, nothing else. We went to a tiny room, hardly larger than a closet, which was equipped with an oxygen outlet and suction. We used neither of these.

This child was obviously quite ill. Skillfully directed by Dr. Cullen, I started a gradual drip of Vinethene on the gauze mask and held it increasingly closer to the child's face. Soon, the child stopped fussing and the resident surgeon accomplished the puncture of the eardrum, extracted some purulent material, and washed out the ear. My attention was forcefully directed to the airway, but no thought of endotracheal intubation occurred.

We discontinued the administration of Vinethene and observed the child, who awakened very promptly. At this moment, I ran quickly to the nearest facility that would accommodate my intense nausea. The room in which we had performed this procedure was not air-conditioned, had no scavenging or particular explosion-prevention devices. Our monitoring was done by observation only, and the only record made was a brief note in the outpatient chart. Except for the nausea, I had a great feeling of satisfaction. I had actually performed a procedure which was beneficial to a sick patient!

There was one other experience during that portion of my final year in medical school that attracted my interest to the specialty of anaesthesia. I was observing a delivery from the observation balcony. As the child was delivered, the patient created a noise which I now recognize as severe laryngospasm, turned blue, and the obstetrician reacted in disorganized panic. I don't recall who was actually administering anesthesia or have any idea what the anesthetic was, but at that moment in answer to a call, Dr. Harold Carron, then a senior resident in Anesthesia, came into the room, took charge of the situation and converted utter chaos into a peaceful, tranquil and happy outcome.

I had been reared in a very small town (population 1,000) in southwestern Iowa. My youth and teen-age years were divided between this small town and an Iowa farm. My father was a banker until the Great Depression, when he made an overnight transition to day laborer and then grocer. Nothing in my background directed me to medicine, but when the time came to "go away to school," I enrolled in a pre-med curriculum without debate. I went to the state university for financial reasons, I guess, but I really considered no other option. I was an avid fan of the Iowa sports teams, whose progress I followed listening to "Dutch" Reagan's broadcasts. My sisters had also attended this school and there was no reason for me to look elsewhere. I had not the slightest idea of becoming anything other than a general practitioner in a small mid-western town. This was probably the only type of physician I knew. My only knowledge of anesthesia prior to entering medical school was that it was a necessary, uncomfortable, and dangerous accompaniment to surgery.

With each clinical rotation in medical school, I thought the specialty of the moment was what I really wanted to be when I grew up. Dr. Cullen was a very capable teacher. He talked common sense and gave students a great deal of personal attention, emphasizing the useful and practical application of what he taught. Anesthesia was one of my last rotations and these experiences were in my mind as I departed for internship.

As an intern, I remember being very impressed with how frequently I applied the basic principles of circulatory and respiratory physiology that had been clearly conveyed to me by Dr. Cullen. An internship rotation on a newly-created anesthesia service directed by Dr. F. C. Jacobson in Duluth, Minnesota further sparked my interest in this specialty. The practical application of "freshman" physiology and pharmacology, and the immediate results seen therefrom, fascinated me. I recall also that although I enjoyed the operating room environment, I did not like the confinement and discomforts of the sterile surgical approach.

World War II ended during my senior year in medical school, but nearly all medical graduates had a two-year obligatory service in either the army or the navy. During my basic training at Fort Sam Houston, Texas, I registered an interest in anesthesia as a career choice and ended up bound for the 97th General Hospital in Frankfurt, Germany, which was then the headquarters of the European Command of the U.S. Army. In that hospital, I was scheduled to work with Captain Jack Osborn to learn enough to serve as an anesthesiologist in the U.S. Army Medical Corps. During my trip overseas, however, Captain Osborn suffered a gastrointestinal bleed and was returned to the United States before I actually got there.

Upon my arrival, despite my lack of training, I found myself assigned as the Chief of Anesthesia and Operating Room Section in one of the largest army hospitals in Europe. My staff consisted of two certified, registered nurse-anaesthetists and one or two orderlies. I was certainly inadequately trained and quite without sufficient experience to fulfill the job and responsibilities given to me. I was frightened but survived for several months. Then I was relieved by the arrival of Dr. Bill Brewster who had had the luxury of 90 days training in anesthesia at Ft. Ord, California. After a few weeks, I was transferred to the Obstetrical Service and later spent one year in Cardiology at Ft. Sam Houston. Both these clinical experiences stood me in good stead many, many times during the remainder of my career.

An interesting memory comes to mind in that, as Chief of Anesthesia in this large army hospital, I was visited by the Theater Chief Consultant in Anesthesiology, Dr. Henry K. Beecher. I was not aware of the exalted status of Dr. Beecher in the world of anesthesia, but I knew that anybody who was Theater Chief Consultant was an important person. I recall clearly that Dr. Beecher spent a great deal of his time talking to me about some of the troubles of the new specialty of anesthesia and the virtues of my taking residency training in his unit at Massachusetts General Hospital. I recall further that in spite of my obvious ignorance and desperate need for help of any kind, Dr. Beecher never came to the operating rooms during his stay with us.

As I prepared to leave the army, I was so provincial in my thinking that I applied only to the program at the University of Iowa, and was very pleased to accept an offer from Dr. Cullen to do my training in his unit. I remain extremely grateful that my provincial thinking persisted, because I received an excellent personal and professional base for my career.

The faculty at Iowa at that time consisted only of Dr. Cullen and Dr. Douglas Eastwood, who had just completed his residency training. There were approximately ten residents and one nurse-anesthetist. We received some help from senior medical students who were hired to assist with night call and obstetrical anaesthesia on the weekends. Dr. Cullen had initiated this procedure in his early days at the University of Iowa. These medical students were given board and room and were affectionately referred to as the "board job boys." Several of Dr. Cullen's residents received an initial impetus for anesthesia in this way.

During my first year, the faculty was enlarged by the addition of Lucien Morris, who came from the University of Wisconsin. Dr. Morris was a very provocative and informative teacher. I learned much from him and it was valuable to have someone on the faculty who had trained elsewhere.

I retain a great—perhaps pathological—respect for that residency program. Located in a small town in the midwest, it was a national leader then and remained so for many years.

It is irresistible to compare the world of anesthesia now and in the early 1950s. Physician personnel were extremely scarce. Few anesthesia residency programs filled and many of those that did accepted all comers without exercising much in the way of selection. Faculties were quite small and it was not uncommon that a department would have only a chief to supervise the training and practice of the entire department. Research was done on a catch-as-catch-can basis, usually in borrowed laboratory space and with meager funding from private donors or related industry. Clinical teaching by the few available faculty was intense and this appeared to be their most important activity. I recall that Dr. Cullen was in the operating room every day and spent a majority of his time in active teaching.

The equipment used was very simple and straightforward. It is interesting to recall that all needles were hand-sharpened, autoclaved, and re-used. Rubber gloves were checked for leaks and patched with bits of rubber. Three-way stopcocks were few in number. They were metal with rubber connecting tubing. We personally cleaned and autoclaved our own three-way stopcocks and guarded them with our lives because the supply was extremely limited. Endotracheal tubes were not used commonly. I have often made the statement to people of this day that, although we had 12 operating rooms to cover, we did not have 12 endotracheal tubes. We would go to the equipment cabinet in the morning and, if our cases weren't at all likely to require intubation, we would not even take laryngoscopes and endotracheal tubes with us. Endotracheal tubes were made of rubber and I don't recall seeing one with a manufactured cuff on it for several years into my career. It was common that uncuffed tubes were used under a mask. We made our own cuffs out of penrose tubing and rubber bands. Again, having made these, we would guard them very jealously. After use, we would take them off the endotracheal tube, wash them, and put them away where only we could find them for subsequent usage.

Monitoring of that day was intense, but certainly seldom electronic. We used blood pressure cuffs on all patients, except for babies and "short cases." I recall that we did not use blood pressure cuffs for tonsillectomies because we were too busy using the suction and holding mouth gags to make marks on the chart. We were taught and admonished to keep a finger on the pulse at all times. Keeping in physical contact was not only important for evaluating pulses, but was alleged to be of some protection against explosions because it prevented static voltage differential from developing between anesthesiologist and patient.

In reality, the drugs we used were also very similar to today's. We had inhalation anesthetics as well as intravenous sedatives, analgesics, and muscle relaxants. The menu of ether, cyclopropane, vinethene and ethylene has been supplanted, and new inhalation drugs have the important difference of being non-explosive. I am not impressed, however, that the inhalation drugs of today have any great advantage. Ether had developed a terrible reputation, some of it earned, but much of it owed to the crude methods used at that time. With the later development of the copper kettle and refinements in the administration of ether, the awareness of patients and, I believe, the nausea, were much reduced.

The narcotics administered at that time were largely morphine and demerol. The change to today's drugs represents valuable fine tuning and provides increased flexibility. It seems to me that the pharmacology is otherwise not much different. We had great results with nitrous-narcotic techniques in the 1940's. Muscle relaxants were essentially limited to curare and gallamine. The philosophy behind the use of relaxants was different, however. Dr. Cullen continually admonished that relaxants were to be merely a *supplement* to real anesthetic agents and were not to be used to mask otherwise suboptimal anesthesia. Antagonists and reversal agents were available, but were used sparingly. We were taught that if one had to use reversal agents, such as neostigmine, this was prima facie evidence that we had overdosed the patient. We were brainwashed with the idea that neostigmine was an *extremely* toxic drug and was to be used only with great caution. I did not personally use reversal agents on a patient until the late 1960's!!

We devoted much attention to the flammability and explosion hazard of the anesthetics of that day. Practices to reduce production of static electricity were numerous. Rules regarding conductive footwear and static-producing nylon hosiery were universal. Intercouplers devised to keep patient, anesthesia personnel, and OR table at the same potential varied from complex commercial devices to simple wet towels placed from patient to table to floor. Conductive flooring was mandated. I recall a new floor placed in our remodeled operating rooms which turned out to be soluble in ether. It was common to spill ether when filling vaporizers and the new floor became a 'muddy' mess. Just prior to my residency, a non-fatal explosion occurred at the University of Iowa that resulted in the rupture of an eardrum of the person administering anesthesia. There was never an explosion involving 'explosive' agents in either department with which I was associated during my career. I was, however, associated with two fatal explosions. Both occurred when "*non-explosive*" anaesthetic techniques were being used. The accidents involved the explosion of bowel gas when electrocautery was used improperly. Whether nitrous oxide contributed was never determined. We used ether anesthesia extensively in rooms that did not have what was considered proper grounding or proper electrical outlets. ENT surgeons routinely operated using a head mirror illuminated by an old-fashioned gooseneck lamp with regular switches not far from the patient's head where we were administering ether in anesthetic concentrations. At the Mayo Clinic, open-drop ether anesthesia was routine for craniotomies in a very large neurosurgical service. Why we avoided explosions is not known, but the problem has been obviated by later developments, of course.

I mentioned that endotracheal intubation was done with rarity. We used endotracheal tubes for all craniotomies and all thoracotomies, and for many airway problems. However, gastrectomies, third-stage thoracoplasties, and most upper belly operations were routinely done without endotracheal anesthesia. It was generally believed that newborns should not be intubate, because it was feared that some edema would develop in the tiny larynx and that airway obstruction would inevitably result. The first two or three anesthetics I administered to newborns with tracheo-esophageal fistulae were done with a mask on the face and no endotracheal tube. This was, of course, essentially an open thoracotomy procedure, and the simultaneous maintenance of adequate anesthesia and adequate respiration was a tremendously difficult task. I am happy to have had that challenging experience, but would not like to have it again. It was considered a triumph if one could leave the operating room still on friendly terms with the surgeon.

Most of our sparing use of endotracheal tubes, either in the operating room or post-operatively, was mostly the result of strenuous objections by our surgical colleagues. There was great fear that endotracheal tubes caused severe damage to the larynx. Our desire to use tubes was thought by some surgical colleagues to be due to our laziness and unwillingness to work to maintain the airway by more conventional means. It is interesting now to note a complete turnaround.

Obstetrical anesthesia, at that time, was certainly given short shrift. I have often thought that the increased incidence (or alleged increased incidence) of vomiting and aspiration in obstetrical anesthesia was due more to the personnel administering anesthesia than to the altered physiology and anatomy of the pregnant state.

There were no intensive care units, but there were dedicated postoperative beds and wards. We, as residents in anesthesia, were rather extensively involved in the post-operative care and evaluation of patients. I believe that the involvement was more intense than it is now in spite of the existence of intensive care units, or, perhaps, because of their existence.

A most remarkable difference between then and now is the content of the operating schedules. During my residency, operations for carcinoma of the stomach were common. They are extremely rare today. Similarly, pneumonectomy and pulmonary lobectomy were common then and now are uncommon. Tonsillectomy and hysterectomy, unusual today, were daily staples then. Conversely, there were no organ transplants or open-heart surgery. Intracranial neurosurgery did not provide experience with vascular malformation; vascular surgery was comparatively nonexistent. The ophthalmologist has extended his repertoire and taken giant steps in prevention of blindness. The obstetrician has new areas of activity in management of fertility problems. The above incomplete list provides examples of new areas of surgical activity, as well as improved technical capacity. It is not readily apparent that we in anesthesia have expanded the scope of our field, though we have improved our techniques and procedures.

At the end of my residency, there were a great number of positions available, in both the academic world and private practice. I, like others, received many of these offers, but my provincialism persisted and I accepted Dr. Cullen's invitation to remain at the University of Iowa. I was offered the salary of approximately $4,000 a year, which was about 15-20 percent of what one could have earned with almost any of the outside offers.

Because less than ten years earlier I had been doing hard manual labor for 20 cents an hour, the thought of $4,000 per year did not seem punitive to me, and I was proud to be selected by Dr. Cullen. As a matter of happenstance, the Veterans Administration Hospital opened on the University of Iowa campus at that time. I was appointed Chief of Anesthesia there and my salary rose to $6,000. This financial bonanza was gratefully received.

My good friend, Jack Moyers, joined the faculty one year before me and we have maintained a friendship that began way back in high school and continues to this day. I am certain that much of what I have learned I acquired from Jack, who was then, as now, a great teacher.

In the mid-fifties, the faculty grew and the responsibilities of the department broadened. The addition of the Veterans Administration Hospital brought new size and new resources. We were able to firmly establish research programs and had time to devote to non-operating-room teaching. We were more successful in recruitment and our faculty increased to perhaps as many as five or six in the next few years. We were embarking on what turned out to be a very bright period in the development of anesthesiology.

I attended my first American Society of Anesthesiologists (ASA) meeting in Washington, D.C., in the autumn of 1951. It is interesting to recall now that the entire meeting, including exhibits, was held in the relatively small hotel (now enlarged) at 16th and K Streets in Washington, D.C. I believe this was then a Sheraton, but later became the Capitol Hilton. Nationwide, the anesthesia fraternity was small and it seemed that everybody knew everybody else.

It was a real eye-opener to me to meet people from other departments and other parts of the country. I was amazed at the differences that existed concerning the preference for one agent versus another or one technique versus another. It was shocking to me that concepts which I had been taught were quite wrong were being used satisfactorily elsewhere. I had an exhibit at the meeting on the use of three-dimensional slides to teach regional anesthesia techniques. I have a painful memory of severe criticism of the exhibit by Dr. F.A.D. Alexander, a reputed expert in regional anesthesia. It was not much of an exhibit by today's standards, but it was an interesting step in my career.

A bit of excitement at that meeting, for me, occurred one evening when I was hurrying up the back stairs as a shortcut to my hotel room and ran into Dwight David Eisenhower, fully dressed in his five-star uniform. He was being recalled to service as the Chief of NATO, as I recall.

I also remember the difficulty in finding funding for this trip. Dr. Cullen had to go hat in hand to the chairman of the Department of Surgery. The surgeon was happy to fund my trip, but emphasized the department limits on food expense. We were not to spend over $6 per day for meals!! This seems like a pittance now, but at that time did provide one with at least adequate nourishment. Certainly, none of us lost weight on any of those sojourns. Compared to now, it was a bit unusual for junior faculty to travel very far or very often.

Research developed along the lines of evaluating drugs, testing equipment and looking for incidence of complications. Certainly, research was simple by today's standards. I came to believe then, as I do now, that the major value of research in a clinical department such as ours was the mental discipline it developed in trainees. We were able to develop interesting questions and made serious attempts to evaluate them. Research of some sophistication was being done on the toxicity of anesthetic agents and the site of action of some intravenous barbiturates.

My own research interests directly followed my clinical interests. Early in my career, I observed that many of the problems of postoperative patients were very similar to ones we encountered daily in the operating room. I refer especially to the development of inadequate respiration, airway obstruction, and problems of maintaining blood pressure and circulatory adequacy. This was especially obvious to me during the severe poliomyelitis epidemics of the late forties and early fifties.

For the patients with poliomyelitis, we immediately recognized the need for and advantage of tracheotomies, but it was unbelievably difficult to get this concept across to the pediatricians and internists who were caring for these patients. We were admonished that "if we really took good care of the patients and had very good nurses," tracheotomies were not necessary.

My first real institutional argumentative role was campaigning for prophylactic tracheotomies in polio and tetanus patients. The resistance was bitter and persistent. The iron lung, or tank respirator, had acquired some popularity among physicians, but was really a terribly poor tool for acute respiratory care. The rigid walls and tank-like nature of this machine sequestered patients rather effectively from adequate nursing care and physician evaluation.

I developed a specific interest in the subject of atelectasis, which had been considered a common accompaniment of the postanesthetic state. The widespread teaching was that *all* atelectasis was secondary to obstruction of airways, with distal absorption of gas. With this belief, we of course applied negative pressure (suction) to the airways to remove obstructing plugs or secretions rather than considering "inflationary" therapy. We later developed the idea that the plugs and obstructions could be, and often were, actually secondary to atelectasis that occurred as primary collapse in quiet lungs. I recall the negative response of surgeons when I prepared a talk for surgical grand rounds, suggesting use of positive pressure, rather than so much negative pressure. I've tried to remember my crushed feelings when I later dealt with younger doctors who presented me with ideas that challenged beliefs I had held over some time. I hope that I was at least partially successful in encouraging their ideas and not crushing their enthusiasm.

In 1956 or 1957, the interest in "inflationary" respiratory care brought me my first contest with hospital directors. I believed something like today's ICU would be beneficial and I spent many hours trying to develop such a unit. We eventually started a very small one, which, as I recall, had room for three or, at most, four patients. We had some impressive success with early patients, so the idea began to grow and development continues to this day. The interest of anesthesiologists in this area was intense for a while, but rapidly declined.

This area of interest advanced my career and enabled me to meet colleagues from many areas of the nation. The group at Massachusetts General Hospital, when they properly investigated these matters, "proved" that atelectasis resulted from a quiet lung, without the necessity of proximal airway obstruction. They popularized the need for and value of a sigh. Positive end-expiratory pressure (PEEP) and continuous positive airway pressure (CPAP) developed from those exchanges with Myron Laver, Henrik Bendixen and Henning Pontoppidan. During my visits and conversations with the Boston group, with whom I shared this common interest, I was happy to re-establish my acquaintance with Dr. Beecher.

This national experience and exposure, combined with the shortage of academic anesthesiologists, led to many very attractive offers of employment elsewhere. In the early 1950's, it must be remembered that there was essentially no open-heart surgery. Dr. Al Blalock had established a solid reputation and considerable public notoriety in the area of repair of congenital heart disease as the developer of the "blue baby operation." He was Chief of Surgery at Johns Hopkins and his operative procedure to bypass pulmonary circulatory obstruction was dramatic in its concept, technique, development, and results. Dr. Blalock was quite famous for his success in this area. You can imagine my feelings when, one morning in 1955, without prior notice, I found myself answering a phone call to hear, "Dr. Hamilton, I'm Al Blalock and I want you to come to Baltimore."

I now think this produced more fear than any other emotion. I viewed the invitation as something like a royal command performance and went to Baltimore three times before eventually deciding to remain at Iowa. Retrospectively, I'm rather certain that thoughts of big city living, sending our children to private schools, and perhaps other provincial fears, were most important in my decision. I recall being offended when Mrs. Blalock inquired as to whether television had yet made its way to Iowa. Further conversation revealed that we had more television channels available than she had in Baltimore at that time. Dr. Blalock was very kind to me and I was convinced that he was seriously interested in the development of a proper professional department of anesthesiology in his school.

A most interesting aspect of this episode was the correspondence I received from many senior anesthesiologists throughout the eastern and central United States. They advised me to avoid the position at Johns Hopkins because Blalock was reputed to be strongly against physician anesthesia. The failure of anesthesia to develop there was said to be his fault. Therefore nothing good could ever happen there. It was never clear to me how these detractors thought that anesthesia would ever develop in this very important educational institution if someone didn't go there and take the job. This was probably my first exposure to the national tendency of our specialty to blame others—usually surgeons and hospital administrators—for our inability to develop the respect and status we desired.

In truth, Dr. Blalock was not opposed to physician anesthesia and I was convinced that he would be a valuable supporter of someone who took the job seriously and developed the specialty. Dr. Don Benson, who did take the job, confirmed this opinion on many occasions. It is of further interest that Dr. E. M. (Manny) Papper, whom I had met but knew only superficially at that time, was the only one in the United States who encouraged me to take this position. He, apparently alone, saw this as a great opportunity in a great institution that needed someone to step in and develop the specialty properly. I believe Manny was correct. I also believe I was not the one to do this. I was not sufficiently trained or experienced in the realities of the world to take this position and handle it well. It was an experience, however, that led to a profitable interchange with Dr. Papper, and we became colleagues and associates in many activities in later years.

I presented my first paper nationally at the ASA meeting in Seattle, in 1952. Dr. Cullen had obtained a new narcotic antagonist from Hoffman-LaRoche. We administered the combination of rather large doses of demerol with its antagonistic derivative in the hope that something of the narcotic action would be left unantagonized, while respiratory depression was antagonized. Nitrous oxide, of course, needed something to help it provide adequate anaesthesia, and it was our hope that this mixture might provide us a supplement that did not forster respiratory depression to the same degree that narcotics alone did.

I was a newcomer in the field and Dr. Cullen had written the abstract for me. I was quite surprised when I arrived in Seattle, picked up the program, and found out that I was alleged to have discovered many things that I had not discovered at all. I was a bit frightened, but somehow survived this ordeal and I guess the audience was not sufficiently sophisticated to perceive what a bad job I had done. It was really a rather pleasant experience.

The founding and growth of the Association of University Anesthesiologists (AUA) was important in my career. It was originally a small and elite society which fostered my acquaintance with neighbors and colleagues at the Mayo Clinic and the Universities of Minnesota and Wisconsin. The interchange we developed was helpful to all of us. I was extremely proud to be elected to this group in the cold winter of 1956, in Rochester, Minnesota. The entire group was small and I found it exciting and gratifying to meet the "famous" of the specialty. Many names that I held in awe became relatively well known to me. In all of these experiences, I was aided and abetted by the totally unselfish acts of Dr. Cullen. He encouraged, introduced, fostered, and comforted me through these developmental years. He never "did" things for me, but suggested some things to do and provided some time and facilities for me to do them.

Many research techniques were crude and difficult. As examples, the measurement of anesthetic and respiratory gases in the gas or blood phase was quite laborious and, without very skilled help, results were of questionable accuracy. I recall clearly the strong desire to be able to measure pH in body fluids, but this was not available for several years. Without measurements, we were taught some things which seem a bit ridiculous in today's world. For example, I was taught that the normal pH was 7.4 and it varied narowly between 7.38 and 7.42. Variations outside the range of 7.35 to 7.45 were believed nearly fatal. We were never taught the intricacies of pulmonary ventilation/perfusion (V/Q) mismatch because without easy and accurate methods to measure oxygen and carbon dioxide levels in venous and arterial blood, we weren't aware of the variations from theoretic normal that occur so commonly.

There was bitter disappointment in a study I attempted regarding post-operative atelectasis. I eventually abandoned this investigation, designed to determine the frequency of shunting within the lung, because I kept finding low oxygen and low carbon dioxide content in the same blood sample. I knew that intrapulmonary shunting would cause hypoxia but assumed it must also be associated with hypercarbia. The different kinetics of transport of these two gases related to their dissociation characteristics were unknown to me. I thought our laboratory was making incorrect determinations and that the results I was getting were impossible.

When oxygen and carbon dioxide electrodes became available and our understanding of V/Q mismatch developed, I realized how naive I had been. I was at least two or three years late in completing this study. Those concepts, which seemed complex and exciting at that time, now are readily accepted and understood by beginners as obvious and rather mundane.

The measurement of such simple things as pressure in the respiratory or circulatory system was also difficult. Direct blood pressure was measured by attaching an arterial line to a U-tube mercury manometer. A float on the mercury column registered on a smoked drum kymograph. The joys of trying to smoke such a drum evenly and without creating a real mess I remember clearly. Later, ink writers were substituted, and still later, electronic transducers were adapted for this use.

The first such transducers were known to us as strain guages. These were about five inches or so in length and one inch or more in diameter. They had a plastic dome with attachments for three-way stopcocks and catheters. The dome was removed for cleaning and sterilizing and, like everything else, was reusable. Early models required difficult manipulation to balance a Wheatstone bridge. Calibration was not stable and had to be repeated frequently. Noncompliant tubing, which would give a faithful pressure recording, was not readily available. In the cardiac catheterization laboratory and the operating room we actually used lead tubing, which was somewhat malleable and certainly quite non-compliant. The decrease in size and increased ease in use of this instrumentation has been a pleasant evolution to observe. I strongly suspect that the inconveniences of laboratory techniques and procedures discouraged many budding investigators of that day.

Anesthesiologists were interested in anesthetic toxicity, pharmacokinetics, and the circulatory and respiratory effects of new drugs. Statistical analysis was forced upon us. I never mastered statistics but, as I realized their importance and necessity, I always found someone available who could do the statistics in research planning and operation.

I did have an intense interest in better methods of measurement and spent considerable time working with Dr. Jim Elam exploring rapid methods of carbon dioxide analysis in the gas phase. Jim knew Max Liston and we received an early model of the Liston-Folb Infrared CO_2 Analyzer. This later became well known as the Liston-Becker. I recall with embarassment the day when we thought the bugs were sufficiently removed from this apparatus to allow us to show it off to the Surgery Department research seminar. We proudly demonstrated nice curves when tidal breathing was analyzed. This was fine until someone in the audience asked about the effect of water vapor and demonstrated that a similar signal could be produced by bubbling room air through warm water into the meter. It pains me to watch countless uses of this methodology in later years without recognition of the discomfort we experienced in its development.

Jim Elam, with this meter and other gadgets, designed the CO_2 absorbers used in most anesthesia machines in this country today. In these studies, he was aided and abetted in no small degree by the engineering talents of Dr. Elwyn Brown. Interestingly enough, Elwyn Brown and I had worked together—he was my boss—amomg the shelves of the University of Iowa Library, back in pre-war years.

By the last half of the 1950's, my own situation had developed rapidly. Residents were more plentiful and we had sufficient faculty to allow proper time for a real academic life. The morale in the department was high. I was promoted to Associate Professor and moved into a brand new house which cost $31,000. I was then being paid $8,500 a year and thought that I could probably replace my 7-year-old Ford coupe the next year.

We had a vintage era in resident recruitment. From one group, Ted Eger, John Severinghaus, Cloid Green, Jerry Miller, Ernie Guy, Jack Williams and a few others had very interesting and productive later careers. The very productive and continuing association of Severinghaus and Eger started then. I recall a very animated discussion of uptake and distribution which occurred in one of our weekly anesthesia seminars. Seymour Kety had published two versions of his concepts of anesthetic uptake and distribution, and Dr. Charles Pittinger led a seminar based on these writings and his own studies of the uptake and elimination of xenon done at Brookhaven Laboratories, using some new radioactive assay techniques. Charles and I disagreed rather seriously on the similarity, or lack thereof, of uptake and elimination phases and this animated discussion initiated or at least encouraged Eger's interest, which was nurtured by Severinghaus' creative and nimble mind. What a productive evening this was.

The association with Ted provides many memories. As an example, he reasoned that since rubber was pervious to carbon dioxide, we could pass expired gases through lengths of thin rubber tubing and this would allow carbon dioxide to escape and would obviate the need for sodalime which, at that time, was a little bit difficult. We procured what must have been half of the world's supply of Penrose tubing and lined it back and forth on the floor of a large room until the floor was entirely covered. We introduced 5% CO_2 and oxygen at one end and analyzed it as it emerged far downstream, unchanged in content or concentration, after traversing these many, many feet of tubing. Although Ted was disappointed and perhaps a bit embarrassed, I never regarded this as wasted time. He had asked an answerable question and worked to provide the answer. It obviously did not discourage his desire to ask and answer questions in the future.

I'm not sure what started my association with the cardiovascular laboratories of the Department of Medicine at Iowa. I worked as an eager learner under the tutelage of Dr. Jack Eckstein, who was much later to retire from the deanship at Iowa as the senior dean of U.S. medical schools. Jack had been to far-off Boston and learned to think about and measure changes in venous compliance, and to discuss the role of such changes in homeokinesis. Prior to that time, veins were believed by most to be passive conduits. I had been impressed that visible peripheral veins became much larger with the onset of the anesthetic state (regional or general). It followed that if more blood was in the peripheral veins, less must be somewhere else, and that a venous role in the hemodynamics of circulatory changes associated with anesthesia was likely. He was a patient teacher and I learned to think about circulatory alterations and their treatment in a different and more complete manner. I also saw a real benefit in collaborating with other specialties. In spite of efforts, however, I have failed to develop this approach in many of my colleagues. I think our specialty has been ill-served by a rather common practice of isolation.

During this time, I became interested in the treatment of patients with acute tetanus. An interest in this problem was generated during the polio epidemics mentioned previously. Jonas Salk had blessed us by removing polio from our midst, but we still had a persistent incidence of patients with tetanus. Tetanus is a fascinating disease. Its severity varies from almost no symptoms to a fulminating course with death occurring a few hours after the onset of symptoms. This variable course made accurate evaluation of treatment extremely difficult. There could be little question, however, that anesthesia and profound muscle relaxation were needed for the acute and severe spasms that occurred with this disease. The pain was intense and respiration actually ceased during the severe spasms. I often thought it more reasonable to regard this disease as "lockchest," rather than "lockjaw."

The tightly closed mouth was certainly a problem, but most harm came from apnea and hypoventilation. The severe disease lasted for three to four weeks, with a period of residual muscle dysfunction for those fortunate enough to survive. Conventional treatment involved general anesthesia levels of sedation with Avertin fluid or barbiturates. Prolonged circulatory depression, infection and problems of nutrition were tremendous and many patients died. Ventilators were not readily available and certainly were not the efficient machines which we have today. The tank respirators presented the difficulties to which I referred earlier. Position change, skin care, bowel and bladder care, etc., were extremely difficult with these ventilators.

Adequate ventilation was extremely difficult to achieve owing to the tight thoracic cage. The situation cried for use of muscle relaxants (curare and gallamine were the only ones available) and this was tried by many. Success was far from uniform. As I recall, we weren't bothered by hypotension-type problems, despite continuous large doses of the drug for long periods of time, but we were not adequately prepared for care of totally apneic patients—60 minutes of every hour, every day, every week, for the entire three weeks or more.

We also had difficulty in managing those patients who survived to the end of the active tetanus period when we attempted to wean them from the respirator. We had patients who were not strong enough to breathe on their own, but too strong to be ventilated by the inadequate respirators of the day. Our knowledge of reversal agents was primitive and, in fact, downright wrong, and the survival rate continued to be low and the complication rate high. This experience did, however, help us to develop the structure for our intensive care units later.

We had a tetanus team of anesthesiologists and surgeons who were called to actually "babysit" these patients. The long and severe course of the disease, the poorly developed equipment, and the lack of a continuous care frequently combined to defeat us. We were proud of an overall survival rate of 50 percent over a period of a couple of years. I remember being completely convinced that antitoxin was of almost no effect once clinical symptoms appeared. We never proved this, but we repeatedly saw patients deteriorate rapidly in the face of huge doses of antitoxin. I, again, enjoyed our relationship with other departments working on this project, and respiratory care offered me exposure to general medicine which was not part of operating room anesthesia experiences.

With the broadened and exciting clinical engsgrmrnt, new research opportunities and improved resident recruitment as well as a livable wage, the world seemed rosy. I recall discussing this with Jim Eckenhoff, who was then second-in-command to Robert Dripps at the University of Pennsylvania. We concluded that the two of us had the best of all possible worlds, with the opportunities that existed and excellent department chairs to do administrative work. We were convinced that we did not want to be department chairs!! (We later proved ourselves human by accepting department chairmanships that effectively stopped our research careers.)

My happy experience was cut short when Dr. Cullen announced in the autumn of 1957 that he was leaving Iowa for a similar position at the University of California in San Francisco. This announcement x came as a real shock to me. I had never considered such a radical change in my world. Anesthesia was then a division of general surgery at Iowa and I was not aware that this situation had ever been a deterrent to Dr. Cullen. He insisted on departmental status when he went to California and this suggested to me that it must be quite important.

The search committee at Iowa nominated me to succeed Dr. Cullen and I had also been asked to look at the Chairmasnship in Anesthesia at the newly-formed University of Florida School of Medicine in Gainesville. I was still firmly attached to Iowa and the Dean at Florida made my decision easier by never offering me a position there. The thought of succeeding Cullen was most frightening. I was certain that no one—especially me—could do what he did, but I accepted the position, without departmental status, and a new aspect of my career began.

Today's chairs are quick to tell me how easy I had it then, compared to the terrible problems that exist today. I must have had it easy, since I survived and succeeded, to some extent. I enjoyed it all the way. Today's problems are new and tough, but in 1958 and the years immediately following, we had some tough times, too. The thought of someone having a day or so in the week firmly committed to research or other academic pursuits was unheard of. We had 18 operating rooms and the delivery room to service with a faculty of four and a resident crew that became sorely depleted when Dr. Cullen left. I believe we started only four new residents at that time. The budget was extremely limited and controlled by the Department of Surgery. We were finally able to get Charlie Pittinger some lab time, but it was precious little and parsimoniously funded. Charlie, Jack Moyers, and Leo DeBacker worked endless hours to help us survive.

We all worked diligently at teaching, with a strong commitment to medical students. We employed a few senior students to help us with our work with pre-operative rounds and night and weekend calls. We employed nurse-anesthetists at the VA Hospital and, somehow, survived. We recruited a couple of faculty from overseas and eventually trained our own. Resident recruitment picked up and life gradually improved.

Faculty recruitment was tough, not only because of our workload, but more so because of our very low pay scale. We were frequently told by candidates for our positions that private practice offered incomes ten times as high as those offered by the University of Iowa. We had no extramural research support and, except for a little drug house money, had no funding for research. This may not have been important in recruitment because most candidates had little, if any, research interest. In reality, it is not important to establish which era was the toughest. Each has had serious problems requiring much work and providing much frustration.

I remained at Iowa as chief for nine years. After the rough start and gradual improvement, our faculty increased to ten. I believed this was as many as one would ever need. Resident recruitment, especially from our own students, was excellent.

We finally obtained our own laboratory space and became a separate department in 1963. We were primary instigators in starting a hospital-wide intensive care unit; we had departmental representation on important college and university committees and we became active in national affairs. Members of the department won medical student teaching awards and we were very proud of our accomplishments at that time.

At this time, a most important development occurred for the specialty nationwide. Dr. Papper took a sabbatical leave of absence from his position at Columbia and spent it at the National Institutes of Health (NIH). I can't recall the exact dates, but he pushed the proper buttons to get research support established for our specialty from the NIH. There were grants for both clinical and research training for faculty, and anesthesiologists were established members with representation on the two NIH surgical study sections existing at that time.

I had an interesting educational opportunity in 1964. The Middle Eastern countries wanted to organize their own anesthesiology society and invited representatives from many countries to attend the formal inaugural meeting. I assume Dr. Cullen had been invited and couldn't attend, so he suggested me. Bernard Branstetter was the professor at the American University of Beirut and knew Dr. Cullen well. At any rate, I was "processed" by the State Department and flew to Beirut where the meeting was to occur. Here, one of the highlights of my professional career occurred. I met and became well acquainted with Sir

Robert MacIntosh from Oxford University. He was probably the best-known anesthesiologist in the world and it was a real thrill to get to know him. I had later opportunities to strengthen this acquaintance. I was also to learn first-hand of the realities of Middle Eastern politics. Several nations would not consider Israel as a member of this society, while others would not condone a Middle Eastern society without Israel. It's not surprising that the meeting broke up without the society's actual formation. It was created later, and I know not what compromises made that possible.

My contacts with other specialties created within me the realization that we in the anesthesiology world needed to seriously upgrade our research activities. Drug testing and simple comparisons of the time were quite pedestrian and most of us didn't know enough to explore the respiratory and circulatory questions which we asked ourselves in the operating room every day. As a result of this realization, and after a bit of inquiry, I obtained support from the National Institutes of Health for a one-year period of research training at the Cardiovascular Research Institute (CVRI) at the University of California at San Francisco. This was under the direct leadership of Dr. Julius Comroe and was a great experience.

I enjoyed meeting new people as well as the release from the frustrating problems of day-to-day departmental administration. The association with Comroe was delightful. He was a wonderful physiologist and perhaps an even better teacher. I remember being very impressed that this man, with all of the talents, qualities and achievements that one could imagine, had genuine inferiority feelings about the role of his laboratory in relation to the clinical departments. Perhaps one needs an inferiority complex to keep driving to the point of such success. The opportunity to spend full time in reading, discussion, and experimentation was well worth the loss of income that I experienced, and was one of the most important and rewarding periods of my life.

After completing this fellowship, I returned to the University of Iowa for five years and was then offered the Chair of Anesthesia at the University of California at San Francisco (UCSF). Dr. Cullen had become Dean of the School and his search committee eventually recommended me for the job. I was torn between my persistent affection for my long-time home in Iowa and its university and the desire to do something new with the attachment to the Cardovacular Research Institute (CVRI). Dr. Comroe was on the search committee that recruited me and greatly influenced my eventual decision. Our daughter actually cast the deciding vote with the comment, "Dad, you've already been here. Do something new!"

A surprise met me upon arriving in San Francisco. I had looked forward to research activities and association with the CVRI personnel. However, I found the department's real need was to strengthen its clinical base. Clinical teaching and operating room coverage had occupied a second priority.

The financial arrangements within the department provided an actual negative incentive for clinical care and left one with limited freedom to recruit. I devoted most of my efforts to correcting these problems and, hopefully, encouraging and developing research at the same time. Owing to Dr. Papper's efforts, anesthesia research center grants were available and we were fortunate enough to receive one at UCSF. This was a real accomplishment that required a lot of work to obtain and a lot of time to maintain and direct.

I spent a good share of my first four years at UCSF developing what I thought to be a proper compensation plan. The existing plan had been devised so that all of the rather generous clinical income was divided up among the faculty. Those old hands got a significantly larger share than newcomers. This had two very bad effects: It created a class distinction which was very difficult for newcomers to accept. Then, if we wanted to do recruiting, all senior people would take a salary reduction since the same departmental income would be spread among more people. We eventually developed a program of pooling the income, paying all people on a somewhat fixed basis and providing a positive dollar incentive for clinical care. It was my belief that the only real reward we had to offer for clinical care was in dollars, while those involved in the special activities of research gained more rapid promotion, honoraria from speeches and writing, and received rewards for their efforts in many other fashions. We were also able to plow back a portion of the clinical income into research. One of my failures at UCSF was not realizing the point where the research division was so well developed that we could remove it from the "back" of the clinical component of the department.

This new arrangement caused some difficulties but, in general, worked quite well. I am extremely proud that the faculty group accepted the difficulties, though it was initially difficult and caused serious problems for some.

I had grown up in medicine at a time when Board Certification was not at all common and represented an immeasurably high degree of status—higher than it does now. Therefore, to have the opportunity to examine for the American Board of Anesthesiology was a great honor for me, and my election to the directorship of the Board in 1962 was extra special. I truly enjoyed the twelve years that I spent on the Board and I believe that I became a better teacher, a better administrator, and certainly a better program director as a result of what I learned while on the Board.

I recall being impressed with the "giants" of anesthesia who were sitting in the boardroom when I walked in there in 1962, after having been summoned to receive notification of my election. In the room were Adriani, Dripps, Papper, Leffingwell, Faulconer, Cullen, Haugen, Barrett, Peterson, Little—people associated with the leadership of our specialty for many years. My joy was unlimited. Elected with me were Bob Patrick and Jim Matthews. The three of us and Dave Little developed a great foursome which enjoyed many professional and social adventures associated with the American Board and its meetings. We were later joined by Art Keats, Bob Epstein, Harry Bird, Don

Benson, Rick Siker, Al Betcher, Jim Eckenhoff, Phil Larson, O. B. Crawford, and Ernie Henschel. The Board was a small group and met twice a year for a week. As a result, we developed very strong bonds which have persisted for these many years. It was a truly wonderful, collegiate experience.

While on the Board we improved the accreditation process enormously and removed several programs that did not perform up to standard. We removed much of the bias from the oral examination procedure. We actively supported the formation of the body which later became the Accreditation Council for Graduate Medical Education (ACGME), and established a much more broadly-based and fairer method of graduate medical education accreditation. We helped prevent the abolition of what is now referred to as a clinical base year. It was our belief that a solid year of clinical experience, *with responsibility*, was a vital base for such fields as Ophthalmology, Radiology, Anesthesiology, etc.

Several ideas which I opposed during my time on the Board have subsequently been adopted. Although we rotated UCSF residents in intensive care, I was opposed to a mandatory period of intensive care unit rotation, but this was enacted soon after I left the Board. I have since seen instances in which two months of poor intensive care unit experience has been substituted for good clinical operating room experience merely to satisfy the Board's requirement. I also was opposed to the mandatory fourth year because I was convinced that many of the departments in the United States did not have the faculty or the capacity to train for an additional year. I especially did not like the somewhat mandated curriculum for residents, because I realized that the rotation through various specialties depended a great deal on the facilities available, and not all programs have all facilities.

There is sufficient flexibility in the menu to allow the situation to work well, but it still seems to me that the program director should be allowed to provide training using the best parts of the facilities available, rather than to have an experience which is less-than-good mandated for the residents in the program. It was and is my belief that much of the motivation for the added mandatory year was a theoretical increase in prestige and the fiscal reward which might result from an additional year of training.

The period of my time on the American Board of Anesthesiology ended in 1974. I am amused now by my recollection of a statement made as Bob Patrick and I exited the room on that final day. One of the remaining members of the Board remarked: "Now that those tightwads are gone, we can live a little better. We'll get our names printed on the stationery and we'll set up a special room for the President."

Bob and I had been raised in a period of economic difficulties for the Board, and I expect we were a bit parsimonious, but I'm not sure that printing one's name on the stationery made much of an improvement in the functioning of the Board.

I continued to represent the Anesthesiology Board on the American Board of Medical Specialties (ABMS), a group composed of representatives from each of the specialty boards. This was a very interesting time. Previously, graduate medical education was under the almost exclusive control of the Council on Medical Education of the American Medical Association (AMA). During my time with the ABMS there was a change to a much wider base, giving the AMA, the specialty boards, the practicing specialties, the medical schools, and the hospitals a combined responsibility for the review, design, and accreditation of graduate medical education in the United States. In addition to this broader-based control, the review procedure was restructured into a much more formal design which provided improved due process and enhanced quality of review. There were interesting politics as the AMA struggled to retain control. In spite of this, the AMA served as the Secretariat for the organization and fulfilled functions that none of the other organizations could handle by themselves.

There were, of course, some troubles. Some specialties thought they were giving up sovereignty to a group and, in fact, this was true, but I think that all eventually agreed that this was beneficial. After a few years, some reorganization was undertaken and the committee emerged as the ACGME (Accreditation Council for Graduate Medical Education). This has worked well and it continues to do so.

Because this change occurred in the mid-70's, it's not surprising that we saw an increased role of the house staff members on these committees. The house staff was represented very capably by some young members of the resident physician section of the AMA. They came to these meetings unencumbered by our previous biases and with all the enthusiasm of youth. It was an interesting experience.

I had the pleasure and privilege of serving on four study sections for the National Institutes of Health. These again resulted from Dr. Papper's sojourn in Bethesda. I was on a training grant committee that had been set up specifically for the specialty of anesthesia. The committee offered and reviewed programs in both clinical and research training in an attempt to provide sorely needed faculty who would have the requisite base for their careers. There weren't many applications for these grants and the committee was rather short-lived, although I don't recall the exactly how long.

I also became chair of a special study section that was established to evaluate grants specifically for the study of acupuncture. After President Nixon's historic visit to China, some of his staff mentioned the use of acupuncture for anesthesia in the operating rooms in China. This was not extensively documented, but did produce a great deal of interest in the professional and the public arena. Specific funds were set aside to study this matter and a number of departments applied for them. As a result, this special study section was formed. As I recall, there weren't many valid applications, and few of them were funded. Even fewer results of value were ever obtained. I have never seen a follow-up of this matter; it would be of some interest to find out how much money was actually granted and what the published results of the studies were. We had rejected applications from some prestigious institutions, for which we earned considerable local criticism.

I also served as a member of the Surgery-A study section for a period of four years. This was one of two study sections devoted to the evaluation of proposals related to the discipline of surgery. On each of these, there was one anesthesiologist. I recall that several of the leaders in our specialty were loudly of the opinion that we should have our own study section at the NIH. The number of grants actually awarded to anesthesia departments was quite small and many persons in anesthesia believed that this was because surgeons would not give us proper consideration. My experience told me this was, in fact, not true. Few applications were actually coming from anesthesia departments and surgeons were more than fair in their evaluations. I believe they bent over backwards to be generous in their evaluation of the anesthesia applications they did receive.

The two surgery study sections were later reorganized and one was categorized as Surgery, Anesthesia, and Trauma. I served a period of two years as the first non-surgeon chair of that study section. There were two or three anesthesiologist members of this study section and, again, I believe that anesthesia grants were hampered only by the inadequate number and quality of the applications received from the anesthesia departments. We were certainly treated fairly.

At UCSF, my job became increasingly one of administration, with less and less time available for actual operating room anesthesia. I insisted on spending some time in the operating room, and to the day I quit as chair in 1983 I spent at least two full days in the operating room and took my regular turn at night and weekend call. I firmly believe that this is a very important—in fact, essential—aspect of a clinical chair's duties. With the development of our new financial plan, our department immediately started to grow, because recruitment was greatly facilitated. Each of the faculty had more time available to pursue things which are commonly called academic activities. I'm afraid I never developed a proper plan to keep people from abusing this system, in which some individuals were given time for academic activities but did nothing creative.

I soon learned, with a larger department and a very talented faculty, the importance of delegating tasks. In my early days, the chief of a department did everything. I had found it difficult to believe there were colleagues who would take over large tasks in the department with enough desire, intensity and direction. The hospital chiefs of service in our various hospitals were excellent, and it was not difficult for me to delegate the entire activity to them. In the units within hospitals, however, it was often very difficult for me to keep a proper distance from the resident recruitment, running of the operating room, medical student teaching, etc. That was a continual source of frustration, although we did succeed in all of these areas.

I am proud of the fact that our relationship with the surgeons had been excellent and there were no major complaints. We also had excellent relationships with hospital directors. Robert Derzon, who left us to become the first director of the Health Care Financing Administration (HCFA), was a vigorous and active director of the hospital, but was certainly reasonable and responsive to well-presented ideas. Bill Kerr, who succeeded him, soon achieved a leadership position in the fraternity of hospital directors throughout the United States and was extremely helpful to the Department of Anesthesia. These people are well aware that helping a service as basic as Anesthesia can only help the hospital in its overall function. I don't think that many of them are unwise enough to believe that by crippling Anesthesia, they could benefit the hospital.

Our relations with the medical school were also quite satisfactory. Of course, when I first arrived at UCSF, Dr. Cullen was the dean, and this was a very special association. We got on very well and I'm sure he never gave us any special treatment,. We were always treated fairly during his reign. I didn't do so well with his successor, probably as a result of my own inability to demonstrate to him the role that the Department of Anesthesia played in the school. The departments of Medicine, Pediatrics, and Obstetrics, and to some extent, Surgery, received many more important medical school committee appointments, received more of the critical space allotments, and received more basic faculty support than we did.

I have no argument with Medicine, Pediatrics, Surgery, and Obstetrics having a bigger share of medical education as their responsibility than does a specialty like Anesthesiology. I do believe, however, that today's events support the view that this school would be better off if they had earned their own way and had kept the *practice* of medicine as a more honorable and proper portion of their activities.

In 1975, I took a sabbatical leave and went to the Nuffield Department of Anaesthetics at Oxford University. This was a wonderful time. I returned to the laboratory where I had worked with Cedric Prys Roberts and Pierre Foêx. We were evaluating the cardiovascular effects of some newly introduced inhalation anaesthetic agents. I renewed my acquaintance with Sir Robert MacIntosh and Harry Churchill-Davidson. These were delightful times and the contact with these leaders, I believe, was extremely good for me.

I was impressed with the relatively unstructured graduate medical education pattern existing in Britain. It differed a great deal from the structured program which our American Board and Residency Review Committee situation created in the United States. I'm not sure that the end result is different, although our training is completed in a shorter period of time and it appears to me they have moved towards a more structured system.

We were able to enjoy Oxford and the Cotswolds, and we traveled in Europe a fair amount. I became acquainted with Crampton-Smith and Stanley Feldman, and these contacts have persisted to this day. I was greatly honored when I was invited to return to Oxford to present the address at the 50th anniversary of the Nuffield Department.

While there on sabbatical, I developed type-B hepatitis. Although I was not seriously ill, and was laid up only for a short time, I thought it was some bad turn of fate that caused this to happen to me while I was on sabbatical. We were not very careful about our own protection in those days and hepatitis was not uncommon among operating room personnel.

In 1978, I was elected Chief of Staff of the University Hospital. I was the first full-time faculty member to hold this position. The increasing role of outside forces was already showing its face at that time. For instance, for the first time, we were not allowed to use faculty membership as a criterion for staff appointment to the University Hospital because it might be unfair to patients who were receiving Medicaid. The increased documentation and paperwork necessary to satisfy insurance companies and government agencies who were paying the bills for clinical care were creating problems throughout the hospital, problems which were very keeping us very busy. Also, the Joint Committee on the Accreditation of Hospitals was becoming more aggressive in its review.

We were just beginning to contract with Kaiser and duties as chief of staff were more vigorous than had been advertised when I accepted the job. However, it was a good experience and it began my interest in medical school administration in a serious way. In the academic year 1982-83 I had my 60th birthday, and completed 25 years as a department chair, and one of the residents graduating in that class was the son of one of my former residents at the University of Iowa. The summation of stimuli provided by these events made me think seriously about what to do with the remainder of my career. The final decisive factor came about when I looked at the chairs of other clinical departments in our school and realized that we were all of a similar age. I was well aware of the shortage of resources at the school, and thought I would be doing my successor and the Department a favor if I were to be first out, thereby placing the Department first in line for the very limited resources. I think this proved correct.

About this time, I had been on the short list for a few deanships in the western part of the United States, but I was always a bridesmaid and never a bride. I was on the list at UCSF in 1983. Dr. Rudi Schmid, who was offered and accepted the position, then offered me the job as Vice-Dean of the School of Medicine and Associate Dean for Clinical Affairs. This offer came soon after I had resigned from the chairmanship and seemed to me to constitute a great opportunity. I had developed an interest in medical school administration and it seemed wise to assume a position which would take me out of the way of my successor in the Department.

I spent nine years in the Dean's Office. I continued my operating room duties one day a week, as well as regular night call, for seven years and, with this to keep me in touch with my old friends, I enjoyed the change of scene. During my deanship, I spent a lot of time organizing the clinical faculty into a clinical practice organization. We saw the need for a unified approach to contracting and dealing with the outside forces of the changing world. I believe this time was very well spent and has proven very beneficial in the activities that have followed. I was also in charge of house staff affairs and I enjoyed my continuing activities and contacts with graduate medical education. The final two years, I did no operating room work and worked only four days a week in the Dean's Office. The perennial three-day weekend was increasingly attractive and I retired completely in July 1992.

During my last two years in the Dean's Office, one major effort was a merger with Mt. Zion Hospital, a major community hospital in San Francisco. This merger was an early one of many that have occurred in San Francisco, and elsewhere in the nation, in response to the changes in the health care financing of this time. At UCSF we had a terrible shortage of space and increasing space on our campus being limited by the activist nature of the neighborhood. The only way we could make changes that would allow us to develop new programs and strengthen existing ones was to join with another hospital.

I have been retired for four years and I still return to the department one day per week, which I spend in the operating room with a resident. I really savor the continued contact with the department, of which I am very proud. I enjoy the brief socializing with former colleagues in the lunchrooms. Like all old-timers, I'm discouraged by the trend to automation with less detailed clinical attention to patients, but I freely admit that patients are obviously receiving excellent and safe care. My frustrations are perhaps my failure to adapt to the new world. The residents are polite enough to tell me they enjoy communicating with me, and I have a clear understanding with Dr. Miller that he will fire me when I become incompetent, which I inevitably will.

After something in excess of 50 years of personal experience in anesthesia, it's inescapable that I be asked to make comparisons between then and now, and to identify the meaningful changes that have occurred. Perhaps the greatest accomplishments are those in concept and generalities. Anesthesia is no longer a major risk factor in surgical therapy or surgical decision-making. It's been years since I've seen or heard of a patient being denied needed surgical therapy because of a lack of capacity to "survive the anesthetic." Factors which were *contraindications* to surgery have now become *indications* for extensive anesthetic and surgical intervention. I believe anesthesia has made a large contribution to this change.

Anesthesia is now broadly perceived by the informed world as an anti-stress, rather than a stress, per se. Additionally, patients now visited preoperatively never immediately shrink back and say, "You're not going to give me ether, are you?" Seldom do we meet patients who withdraw from us in fear. Many are properly concerned with risks and have appropriate questions and desires, most of which can be satisfied. The experiences that patients have with anesthesia are not remembered as unpleasant. This is a real gain for society.

Anesthesia is now well represented on hospital staff organizations and in medical school structures. That improved status is now attainable by all who earn the respect of their colleagues. This standing did not obtain in the late forties and early fifties, and it is a tremendous improvement.

I am immensely pleased with and proud of "my" residents. I hear from several who are leaders in their hospital communities and their state and national medical societies. Many have achieved success in academic halls and very few have failed. I am proud of all of these people and of the contacts that I maintain with them.

I end my professional career with many satisfactions, as recalled above, but with serious concerns for the specialty. We have not kept up with research and expansion of knowledge in our own and related disciplines. We were and remain late in encompassing molecular and cellular biology. The evaluation of emerging anesthetic drugs that vary in minor ways from existing agents is not exemplary university research. I perceive that we are beginning to change, but we are still far behind.

We have not expanded our overall role or activities in the practice of medicine and do not compare favorably in this respect with fields such as transplant surgery and medicine, advances in oncology, and treatment and prevention of cardiovascular disease. Interestingly, we did start to expand in several areas, such as inhalation therapy, blood banking, intensive care, emergency resuscitation, and treatment of pain. We had good reason and background to develop in these areas, but in each instance we withdrew to the familiar and more comfortable confines of the operating room.

The reasons for our failure to grow and develop in these areas are many. The operating room practice is confining and impedes outside activities. We were very well paid for our regular practice and other activities encroached on this. The changing environment of 1996 may alter the situation and favor or hinder our growth in other areas. Many leaders in Anesthesia share the concerns expressed here and are working to improve these matters.

There is hope that the current renewal of interest and activity in pain and pain therapy will succeed in breaking the pattern this time. This appears to be a fertile field for research, yet I have some concern about our ability to maintain a distinct practice based on a single symptom in patients who will initially have consulted someone else.

It has been a huge pleasure to be part of this developmental era in our specialty. I wouldn't trade my university career for any that I can imagine. I've had the special privilege of working at two very fine universities and developing associations with wonderful groups of people. I am proud to maintain those relationships to this day.

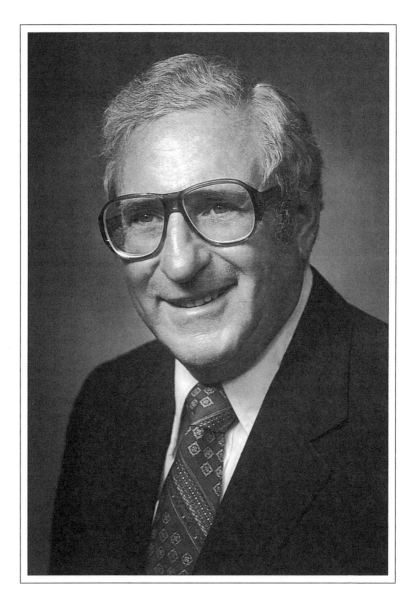

Eli Brown, M.D.

AN AUTOBIOGRAPHICAL ESSAY

ELI BROWN, M.D.

History is the essence of
innumerable biographies
— Thomas Carlyle

AN AUTOBIOGRAPHICAL ESSAY

When I was asked to write my biography, I hesitated for the same reason that I hesitate to show photographs of my travels. However, on reflection, I remembered that Carlyle wrote, "History is the essence of innumerable biographies." With that thought in mind, I embark upon the project in the hope that my experiences might contribute in some small part to the history of anesthesiology. To provide a proper perspective, it is necessary that I start with a brief background of events prior to my becoming an anesthesiologist.

I was born in the early morning of April 25, 1923 at Mercy Hospital in Baltimore, Maryland the fifth of six children. The early years of my life were not particularly unusual. I attended elementary and high school in Baltimore and I was admitted to the University of Maryland in 1940. Even though, I pursued a balanced study of arts and sciences at college, I was inevitably drawn to the study of medicine. My decision to enter the field of medicine was undoubtedly influenced by the environment of my home. My brother and two brothers-in-law were physicians, my oldest sister was a bacteriologist and another sister was a nurse. After completing three years of undergraduate studies, I was admitted to the University of Maryland School of Medicine.

Although I was not aware of it at the time, my path toward a career in anesthesiology probably started in medical school. The two teachers who greatly influenced me were Dr. E. A. Uelenhuth, Professor of Anatomy, and Dr. John Krantz, Professor of Pharmacology. Dr. Uelenhuth's emphasis on the importance of dissection to understand anatomy had a strong influence on my eventual interest in regional anesthesia.

Dr. John Krantz had a very engaging style of teaching. Indeed, his course in Pharmacology was known among students as the "hour of charm." He described the origins of anesthesiology in this country in a manner that kept students spellbound. Further, his research with regard to new inhalation agents was equally impressive.

Another event that may have directed me toward the specialty of anesthesiology occurred during a lecture by my Professor of Surgery, Dr. Shipley. I recall vividly his statement that good anesthesia was essential for successful surgery. He said, "If you have two assistants, one very competent and the other mediocre, make the competent physician your anesthetist and the mediocre physician your assistant surgeon." Of course, in those days most anesthetics were administered by nurses, residents or family practitioners.

Upon graduation from the University of Maryland in 1946 I obtained an intership at the Jewish Hospital in Brooklyn, New York. I chose that hospital for two reasons. First, I was interested in pediatrics and Jewish Hospital had an outstanding department of pediatrics and secondly, I was a bachelor and wanted to experience life in the "big city." On my very first evening at the hospital I was assigned to the obstetrical service where I was told to administer anesthesia to a patient who was about to deliver her baby. I was instructed to place the mask on the patient's face and to turn the ether bubbler up to where I could see three bubbles. That was the only instruction I received. Obviously, I was frightened to death. Although I got through the anesthetic and delivery without incident, I immediately decided that I needed to learn more about the administration of anesthesia so I chose an elective on the anesthesia service for later that year. When doing the rotation on anesthesiology, I was impressed by the awesome responsibility of keeping a patient alive and well while providing the surgeon with the necessary conditions to perform his task. Also, I enjoyed the milieu of the operating room even though I had no interest in performing surgery. Accordingly, I applied for and was granted a residency position in anesthesiology under Dr. I. M. Pallin. As residents we were required to attend an anatomy course at the Long Island College of Medicine. We actually dissected a cadaver and identified those structures that were necessary for the appropriate performance of regional anesthesia. This experience reinforced my medical school experience in anatomy and provided the additional background that led to my research and teaching of regional anesthesia. During my residency I read avidly the available literature on anesthesiology because I was reminded of Osler's statement to wit: "It's astonishing with how little reading a doctor can practice medicine, but it is not astonishing how badly he may do it." There were very few books available on anesthesiology. I recall, Dr. Paul Wood pointing out to residents the opportunities available for those who have a talent for writing. Further impetus toward scholarly activity was provided at the Monday evening conferences at Bellvue Hospital with Drs. Rovenstine and Papper. There was usually a very spirited and clinically oriented discussion of case management based upon sound scientific principles.

As a resident and later as an attending anesthesiologist, I recall working with Dr. Rudolph Nissan the renowned thoracic and general surgeon who introduced the fundoplication operation for esophageal reflux. While at Jewish Hospital, Dr. Nissan operated on such notable people as Albert Einstein and the singer Marion Anderson. He appreciated good anesthesia, but for some reason was always concerned about the use of endotracheal tubes. This fact is especially curious for someone who pioneered in chest surgery. When Dr. Nissan left Jewish Hospital he became Professor of Surgery at the University of Basel in Switzerland. It is noteworthy that not too long thereafter Myron Laver, the well-known anesthesiologist from Massachusetts General Hospital, went to Basel Switzerland to assume the chair of the Department of Anesthesiology.

Other interesting experiences during my residency included participation in the use of music to supplement anesthesia with N_2O and oxygen. This technique is now used in many dental offices. One of my co-residents at Jewish Hospital was Dr. Robert Berman. Bob was constantly experimenting with equipment to develop improved methods of administering anesthesia. He developed the Berman Airway and other types of equipment. I met him recently and learned that he continues to invent anesthesia equipment aided by his son who is also an anesthesiologist.

After one year of residency in anesthesiology I was recalled into the army and assigned to Valley Forge General Hospital (VFGH). That was a very fortunate assignment since my anesthesia training was supervised by Drs. Dripps, Dumke and Eckenhoff of the University of Pennsylvania who were the consultants at VFGH at that time. Dr. Dripps invited me to attend the educational sessions at the University of Pennsylvania in Philadelphia. I accepted the invitation eagerly and attended the evening conferences regularly. These outstanding anesthesiologists provided me with "one on one" teaching in the operating room. This experience convinced me that some of the most effective teaching can take place in the clinical setting in the operating room while the resident is administering anesthesia. It is difficult to learn to administer anesthesia without appropriate supervision since one tends to make the same mistakes repeatedly. In a sense it's very much like learning the game of golf. One can play frequently and never improve his/her game, whereas a few sessions with a teaching professional can be very effective.

At VFGH, Drs. Cannon, Blocker and other famous plastic surgeons were performing very complicated facial plastic surgery. Since I did not have the sophisticated equipment now available, it was necessary for me to adapt basic anesthesia equipment to the special needs of this type of surgery. Although it was a difficult task, it helped me to better comprehend many basic principles related to the administration of anesthesia. My task was eased somewhat, however, because Dr. Douglas Sanders of Wilmington, Delaware who preceded me at VFGH left much of the equipment that he invented such as a special laryngoscope and armored endotracheal tubes. After spending a year at VFGH I passed the written examination of the American Board of Anesthesiology.

Following my tour of duty at Valley Forge I was sent overseas to Japan where I became Chief of Anesthesiology at the Osaka General Hospital. During the latter part of 1949 and the early part of 1950 the hospital census was 95-100 patients. Since I was not too busy I had the opportunity to visit some of the Japanese hospitals in Osaka and Kobe. I helped educate Japanese physicians to administer anesthesia and I was able to provide surplus equipment for them to use. With the outbreak of the Korean War everything changed. Many of our staff were sent to Korea. At the time, to my knowledge, I was the only trained anesthesiologist in Japan. There was also only one trained surgeon at Osaka General Hospital, Lt. Colonel Rush. In the first few weeks after the outbreak of the war our census increased six to eight fold. The only patients that we accepted were wounded soldiers from the battlefield. The entire staff of the hospital including dentists were converted into surgical staff and I was compelled to use corpsmen to monitor patients under anesthesia. We used three operating rooms. I would induce the anesthetic and then turn the case over to one of the corpsmen. The surgical staff would open the abdomen and Lt. Colonel Rush would do the definitive work and leave the closure of the wound to the assigned personnel who, sometimes, were oral surgeons or dentists. Our operating schedule began at six o'clock in the morning and we worked until midnight. We made rounds for the purposes of triage and then usually had a few hours of sleep.

We continued to work this way for approximately one month. I do not recall ever working harder than I did during the four weeks before additional surgical staff began to arrive at our hospital. After being rotated back to the United States, I was assigned to Camp Pickett in Blackstone, Virginia. When I arrived I was told that I would not only be Chief of Anesthesiology but also Chief of Radiology. When I asked the Colonel why he chose me as Chief of Radiology he informed me, with typical army logic, that Radiology was located adjacent to the operating room. I served in this dual capacity for approximately a year after which time I was honorably discharged from the army.

Since I wanted to return to my home town, Baltimore, I went to Johns Hopkins Hospital and interviewed with Dr. Robert Hingson. He strongly advised me against practicing anesthesia at Johns Hopkins because anesthesia was held in very low regard by the Chief of Surgery and surgical staff. Indeed, Dr. Hingson told me that he was not allowed to go into the operating room and could only function as an anesthesiologist on the obstetrical service. That type of arrangement did not interest me so I returned to New York and accepted a position on the attending staff at the Jewish Hospital of Brooklyn. The Jewish Hospital was one of the few hospitals in the United States where there was full-time coverage of obstetrical anesthesia by anesthesiologists. Anesthesiologists from many academic centers including Columbia Presbyterian Hospital were recruited to help cover the obstetrical anesthesia service. Dr. Bernard Cappe, Chief of Obstetrical Anesthesia, has never received proper credit for having initiated full-time coverage of obstetrical anesthesia and having established one of the earliest epidural services.

In 1952 I took my oral examinations for certification by the American Board of Anesthesiology at Swampscott, Massachusetts. There is an interesting anecdote regarding the examinations. I entered the room in which Dr. Donald Burdick was the senior examiner. His junior examiner was a physician from New Jersey whose name I have forgotten. I recall that Dr. Burdick asked me about the use of "Efocaine," a long acting local anesthetic. After I answered the basic questions concerning the pharmacology and use of "Efocaine," he asked me if I had ever used the drug for epidural anesthesia. I told him that I had tried it once or twice but it had caused severe burning on injection into the epidural space. At that point, Dr. Burdick turned to his junior examiner and said, "You see, I told you so." I passed the examination and was granted my certificate by the American Board of Anesthesiology. Subsequently, I applied and received certification by the American College of Anesthesiology by reciprocity.

I remained at the Jewish Hospital until 1954, when during a fraternity reunion a physician from Detroit asked if I might be interested in becoming Chair of the Anesthesiology Department in a hospital that had recently opened. Although I had serious doubts about accepting a position in a city known for violent labor disputes and the antisemitism of Father Coughlin, I agreed to visit the hospital. I was very impressed with the beauty of the suburban area, the friendliness of the people whom I met and the opportunity for professional advancement. Also, I was encouraged to accept the position by Dr. Paul Dumke who had recently moved to Detroit to accept the Chair at Henry Ford Hospital. I had a major problem to overcome, however, before I could accept the position. My wife, Estelle, was a professional ballerina. She had danced with the New York City Ballet, the Metropolitan Opera, in Broadway shows and Radio City Music Hall's Corps de Ballet. She gave up her dancing career to raise our children but thought she might return to dancing when our children were older. Furthermore, she was a native New Yorker who believed the adage that "All land beyond the Hudson River is Indian territory." I like to say that "I dragged her kicking and screaming across the Hudson River." The truth is, however, that Estelle was a devoted wife who was willing to sacrifice her career so that I might have the opportunity for professional advancement. In retrospect, the move to Detroit was a very wise decision. Estelle pursued a new career in literature and writing and I attained a stature in anesthesiology and in my community that would almost certainly not have been possible had I remained in New York City.

Sinai Hospital of Detroit had been in existence for approximately a year and a half when I assumed the Chair of a department that consisted of ten C.R.N.A.'s and no physicians. Although the surgical staff was perfectly willing to have me supervise the CRNAs and charge fees for all of the seven rooms they were operating, I refused to do so on ethical grounds even though many other anesthesiologists in the area were practicing in that manner. I charged only for those cases in which I actively participated. Although I was administratively in charge of the Department, I did not receive a salary for that. My goal was to develop a residency program in anesthesiology which required that I recruit a faculty of anesthesiologists. The fact is, however, I never discharged a nurse anesthetist for the purpose of replacing her or him with an anesthesiologist. As the CRNA's resigned for various personal reasons, I replaced them with anesthesiologists. The only two CRNA's that I actually fired were a drug addict and the CRNA who was nominally in charge of the Department prior to my arrival and refused to accept the concept of supervision by an anesthesiologist.

I began my residency program in anesthesiology by accepting two applicants. One was a Canadian medical graduate who entered the first year of training. The second was an American medical graduate who entered the second year of training having served his first year at the Jewish Hospital of Brooklyn. By the year 1959, I had four residents and five attending staff. It's interesting that after I had a staff of five anesthesiologists, every time I wanted to add another anesthesiologist there were loud complaints from those already in the group that it would decrease their income. This is similar to the present circumstance where residents who are completing programs in anesthesiology are unable to find positions even though there seem to be many positions available for CRNAs. Eventually I increased my staff to 20 anesthesiologists. Significantly, all earned a very good income though not the exorbitant income of some of our colleagues who supervised a qreater number of anesthetics with a smaller staff of anesthesiologists. It is unfortunate that the availability of positions for anesthesiologists is dictated by economics rather than quality of care considerations.

By the early 1970s I had a department that was essentially composed of anesthesiologists. There were still two to three CRNAs present but they mostly monitored stand-by anesthetics or relieved residents for conference. I gradually increased the number of residents but I never took more than eight per year. My concept was that I would accept only qualified applicants for residency training. It was difficult to attract residents in the years 1955-75 and many programs accepted unqualified residents in order to maintain service responsibilities. I chose to limit the number of residents and added more staff.

In the 1950s and 60s it was the philosophy of many departments of anesthesiology including some of the very prestigious university departments that residents should be allowed to administer anesthesia on their own so that they "could get experience". In many institutions the residents were permitted to work essentially unsupervised. I firmly believed that making the same mistake a hundred times does not qualify as "experience". Consequently, I insisted upon one to two coverage of our residents as a maximum. When Dr. James Matthews came to site visit our residency he was amazed that we supervised our residents so closely. Before he left Detroit I think he was convinced that our concept was credible. I suggested to the Residency Review Committee that no program should be approved unless there was at least a one to two ratio of attending staff to residents. This concept was finally adopted many years later.

In our residency program all patients were seen by the resident assigned to the case and by an attending physician as well. We had an early morning conference daily in which all residents reported on the physical status and choice of anesthetic of their patients. Each resident's presentation was critiqued by the attending anesthesiologist who visited the patient. Although most of the cases were relatively routine and required little discussion there were always three to five cases that were extremely interesting and controversial so that the meeting was an excellent teaching session. Despite the dearth of available applicants, we had little trouble recruiting excellent residents during the

1970's because Sinai Hospital was the main teaching hospital for anesthesiology of Wayne State University. We participated in the clinical correlation conferences of the Department of Pharmacology for second year students and an elective program for fourth year students. My staff and I were very conscientious in teaching students assigned to anesthesiology. As a result, I received the "Outstanding Clinical Faculty Award" from the students in 1977.

At the same time that I was building my department I became actively involved in hospital affairs. Two years after I arrived I was elected Secretary of the Medical Staff. I continued to serve in that capacity until 1968 when I was elected Vice-Chief of the Medical Staff and five years later I was elected Chief of the Medical Staff. During the years that I was Vice-Chief of Staff I also served as Chief of Medical Education at the hospital. Although this work entailed many evenings away from home, I felt that it was important because it greatly enhanced the prestige of our department. For many years there was a rule in the by-laws of the hospital that no physician could serve as a member of the Board of Trustees. When the prohibition was removed in 1987, I was elected as a member of the Board of Trustees of Sinai Hospital and served in that capacity until 1991 when I left my position as Chief of Anesthesiology. I am very proud that my son, Morris Brown, was appointed to succeed me as Chief of Anesthesiology at Sinai Hospital of Detroit. He has led the Department very effectively and he is actively involved in ASA activities. Morris and I have worked together on a number of research projects, and we are presently collaborating in editing a textbook on Postanesthesia Care.

As Chief of Anesthesiology at Sinai, I had adequate opportunity to visit other departments of anesthesiology as a guest lecturer or site reviewer. On a visit to Toledo, Ohio I had the rare opportunity to observe Dr. Clement administer anesthesia for surgery using nitrous oxide-oxygen anesthesia. It became obvious that the use of the secondary saturation technique was safe in his hands because of his great skill at observing the respiratory signs of anesthesia and his ability to perform "blind nasotracheal" intubation quickly and flawlessly.

WAYNE STATE UNIVERSITY

My association with Wayne State University began shortly after my arrival in Detroit. I began to accept students in 1956. I gradually rose in academic rank from Assistant Professor to Professor in 1973. In 1975, I was asked to assume the chair of the Department of Anesthesiology at Wayne State University. One of the first activities that I initiated was a course in "Anatomy and Techniques of Regional Anesthesia and Pain Management," which is given annually. To my knowledge, this course is the only educational program in the country that includes a laboratory session involving anatomical dissection.

In the early 1950s Wayne State University had an excellent residency training program under the leadership of Dr. Ferdinand Greifenstein. After Dr. Greifenstein left Wayne State University, Dr. Dal Santo who had trained with Dr. Beecher at the Massachusetts General Hospital was appointed Chair of the Department. Dr. Dal Santo made a valiant attempt to advance the academic stature of the Department of Anesthesiology but he was working under very difficult circumstances. The major teaching hospital was Detroit Receiving Hospital, a city facility that admitted mainly indigent patients. Unfortunately, there was not sufficient financial support to retain the type of faculty that was necessary to effectively conduct a teaching program. Consequently, the level of the program gradually deteriorated until there was a loss of residency accreditation in the early 70s. Since there was practically no academic program in anesthesiology at Wayne State University at that time, my department at Sinai Hospital accepted the responsibility for teaching students. Although this increased our workload tremendously, it had the major advantage (as I pointed out previously) of allowing us to recruit some of the best students as residents in anesthesiology. A number of these physicians joined our department as faculty after completing the residency program.

When I was appointed Chairman of the Department of Anesthesiology at Wayne State University, it was my intent to form an intergrated academic department consisting of the Departments of Anesthesiology of Detroit Receiving Hospital, Harper Hospital, Hutzel Hospital, Children's Hospital, and Sinai Hospital. Even though the Dean was strongly in favor of this concept, it was extremely difficult to put the plan into effect. The private anesthesia groups that worked in the various hospitals were not willing to give up their private practice for an academic position. Their stand was supported by many of the private practice surgeons who supported the hospitals by admitting patients. The administrators of the hospital were concerned about losing patients and they were also concerned that the large number of CRNAs who were functioning in anesthesia at these hospitals would all leave abruptly and force a drastic reduction in service to surgeons. In an era of intense competition among hospitals, this was a frightening prospect to shortsighted administrators. In short, everyone supported the concept of an integrated academic department, but each of the players was concerned about his or her own security. Consequently, the integration never really got off the ground particularly since there was not even a coherent integration of the hospitals themselves. Furthermore, no one felt any great urgency about initiating change since I was serving as Chairman of the Department of Anesthesiology both at Wayne State University and Sinai Hospital. The residency program in anesthesiology at Sinai Hospital was considered to be a Wayne State University residency even though it was entirely under the auspices of Sinai Hospital. Although Sinai was a major affiliated hospital with the University, it was not a part of the Detroit Medical Center and still is not. In 1991 I resigned as Chairman of the Department of Anesthesiology at Sinai Hospital, though I still retained my position as Chairman of the Department of Anesthesiology at Wayne State University. However, I informed the Dean at that time that I had been offered a position at the University of Miami during the winter months of the year and that I intended to spend some time teaching anesthesiology there. I agreed to remain as Chairman of the Department at Wayne State University until we could form a basis for recruiting a new chairman. During the time I spend at the University of Miami, I am involved in the educational program for residents. This has been a very rewarding experience for me and continues to be so. I sm still hopeful that I can help to form an integrated Department of Anesthesiology at Wayne State University. This will make it possible to recruit a chairman who will be able to establish the type of department that I believe is appropriate for a medical school of the caliber of Wayne State University.

ASA ACTIVITY

Until I moved to Detroit to assume the chairmanship of the Department of Anesthesiology at Sinai Hospital, I was relatively uninvolved in ASA activity. Within a couple of years after I arrived in Detroit, however, I was fortunate to be appointed as alternate delegate to Mary Lou Byrd who was an ASA delegate at the time. Dr. Byrd was one of Dr. Rovenstine's early residents and practiced at Butterworth Hospital in Grand Rapids, Michigan. She took me "under her wing" and taught me about ASA politics. During the 1950's, Michigan and Wisconsin constituted a single director district and our director at that time was Dr. Bryce Stearns. As our component society grew in numbers we added more delegates. Paul Dumke became a delegate and I became a delegate also. As a delegate I lobbied to divide Michigan and Wisconsin into separate director districts. I succeeded in this endeavor and Dr. Paul Dumke was elected as our District Director. Shortly thereafter, I was elected President of the Michigan Society of Anesthesiology. As I indicated previously, in those days there was a tendency for some anesthesiologists to "supervise" what was known as a "stable of CRNAs." I felt that this practice exploited both CRNAs and patients. I believed that more personal service by anesthesiologists would result in not only better quality of anesthesia care but a more realistic fee structure. Michigan had among the lowest fees in the United States. The very low fees paid by Blue Shield and other insurance companies were justified by them on the basis that anesthesiologists were being paid for multiple anesthetics concurrently. The situation was obviously unfair to those anesthesiologists who administered anesthesia personally and to academic departments who were constrained by the requirements of a teaching program to a maximum of 1:2 ratio. More important, we wanted to exert peer presure on those anesthesiology groups in Michigan who were not extending high quality anesthesia care. We worked to establish a milieu that would attract more anesthesiologists to Michigan and elevate the quality of anesthesia care.

On the national scene, there was some concern that the East and West Coast, particularly New York and California, were dominating the election process in the American Society of Anesthesiologists. Therefore, a number of anesthesiologists from the Midwest led by Dr. Paul Dumke from Michigan and Dr. De Piero from Ohio decided to form a Midwest Caucus. During the early years the Midwest Caucus was a very loosely knit group. As a young delegate I was appointed spokesperson for the group. My job at that time was simply to go out and speak to people from other caucuses particularly New York, California, and other large states such as Texas in order to find out what was going on and to bring that information back to the people at the Midwest Caucus. I was sort of like Tonto in the Lone Ranger radio program. Although I had very little influence, because of my youth and inexperience, the position provided experience for my later activities in the ASA. An interesting incident occurred during an ASA meeting when I attended a scientific session. As I came out the door at the end of the session Dr. De Piero said irately, "What are you doing in there? You are supposed to be getting information about political activities." I apologized profusely for attending the scientific session and pursued my political responsibilities. However, on occasion I was able to "sneak away" to pursue scholarly activity.

During my tenure as delegate, the ABA determined that osteopathic physicians (D.O.) who trained in allopathic hospitals were eligible for certification. Incongruously, these physicians were not eligible for membership in the ASA. I succeeded in getting a resolution passed by the ASA House of Delegates to remove that restriction. I believe that one of my residents, Dr. Stuart Bloom, was the first D.O. to achieve certification by ABA.

Another area of activity in the ASA was the American College of Anesthesiology. I began as a junior Examiner for the American College of Anesthesiology in 1954. In 1968 I was elected to the Board of Governors. Interestingly, I was really not the choice of some of "the powers that be" on the American College at the time. However, people like Paul Dumke and Albert Betcher, who I believe was President of the American Society of Anesthesiologists, were not to be dictated to by a small group as to who was qualified to be elected to the Board of Governors. Accordingly, Dr. Dumke nominated me for a position and I was elected by the ASA Board of Directors for a term on the Board of Governors of the ACA. Once elected, the members of the Board of Governors accepted me graciously. Indeed, within a couple of years I was elected Secretary of the Board of Governors and eventually, Chairman. At a meeting of the ASA Board of Directors at the Marriott Hotel in Chicago, I was having a discussion with Dr. "Pepper" Jenkins, President-Elect of ASA, and Dr. Donald Bridenbaugh, Chairman-Elect of the A.C.A. Board of Governors, in the lobby of the hotel during an intermission. As I looked across the lobby I noticed a young man swoon. I rushed to his side closely followed by my colleagues. We determined that the man was in cardiac arrest so we began cardiopulmonary resuscitation which was successful. At that point, Dr. Joyce Sumner, Secretary of ASA, approached and asked if I would like to administer lidocaine to stabilize the heart. I eyed her quizically and asked where I might obtain the drug. She opened her purse and withdrew a syringe filled with lidocaine which I administered. She told me that she carried the drug in her purse for just such an emergency.

The ACA was at this time a secondary certifying body. Most anesthesiologists were being certified by the ABA. Therefore, it was possible for us to experiment with various innovations such as structured examinations and a "pass-fail" system of grading. Some of the innovations started by the ACA were adopted by the ABA. As the necessity for ACA as a certifying body declined, the Board of Governors sought other means to serve the ASA membership.

Dr. Tom Burnap, a member of the Board of Governors who preceded me as Chair, was a very dynamic person who became interested in Peer Review and Quality Care. During his term as chair he steered the focus of the American College away from its primary role as a certifying body and in the direction of continuing education and Peer Review.

The American College was my introduction into quality care and peer review. I was appointed to the Peer Review Committee by Dr. "Rick" Siker and served on that committee for many years. The Peer Review Committee consisted of a very focused group of people. We were quite far ahead of other specialties with regard to the concept of quality care and peer review. We began with simple guidelines for good anesthesia practice and proceeded on to more specific methods of evaluating quality of care in the various institutions. There was a great deal of resistance to the idea of peer review because many physicians considered it "cookbook practice of medicine" and because of the expense involved in developing quality of care programs. Shortly after my appointment to the committee, I was named Chair of the Peer Review Committee. I appointed people to the committee who had fresh ideas while keeping the core of experienced personnel intact. There were a number of members of the committee who were very much involved in the concept of peer review and it was important to have them continue as members of the committee. However, we did appoint others. One person who comes to mind is Dr. Terry Vitez who had developed a new way of objectively testing for quality care in various institutions. Dr. Vitez brought many new ideas to the committee and introduced us to the concepts of W. Edwards Deming. The Deming philosophy represents a holistic approach for management. Deming views the organization as an integrated whole: it provides a framework for consistent action, is driven by force of quality, and defines quality as a never ending improvement of all processes. We adapted this philosophy to the practice of anesthesiology.

My work with the Peer View Committee inevitably brought me into contact with the Joint Commission on Accreditation of

Hospitals because obviously they were working on standards of care as well. It occurred to me that it was rather odd that the American Society of Anesthesiologists, unlike most other medical specialties, had absolutely no representation at any level of the Joint Commission on Accreditation of Hospitals. I petitioned the Joint Commission for representation on the Professional and Technical Advisory Committee (PTAC) of the Hospital Accreditation program and also for representation on the Ambulatory Care Program. At first, our petition for representation was denied. I proceeded to enlist help from other specialties and from the American Medical Association. Dr. "Pepper" Jenkins who was our delegate to the American Medical Association was very helpful in getting the AMA Commissioners to support our request. Eventually we were granted representation on the PTAC for Hospital Accreditation and Ambulatory Care Accreditation. I was appointed to the PTAC for Hospital Accreditation, and Dr. Harry Wong was appointed to the PTAC for Accreditation of Ambulatory Facilities. At the time that I was appointed to the Professional and Technical Advisory Committee, anesthesiology was grouped with various other service support groups including dietary, respiratory care, and physical therapy. I believe that this was improper and sought a method for getting anesthesiology classified as a clinical medical group along with surgery, medicine, and obstetrics and gynecology. The opportunity to accomplish this goal arose when our committee was seeking ways to integrate the process of peer review in the hospitals. I presented the idea that there ought to be a chapter in the Hospital Accreditation Manual on anesthesia and surgery services which would encompass a peer review process to include surgeons, anesthesiologists, and operating room nurses. The Association of Operating Room Nurses was very supportive of this idea and, because they had a representative on the PTAC, we worked together very closely to have this initiative accepted at the level of the PTAC. Originally the chapter was entitled "Anesthesia and Surgical Services" but, in order to obtain cooperation from the representatives of American College of Surgeons, we had to change it to "Surgery and Anesthesia Services" to which I readily agreed. At about this time I was elected chair of the PTAC which provided me with access to the meetings of the Board of Commissioners of the Joint Commission on Accreditation of Hospitals. After a great deal of negotiation we were finally able to get approval of the chapter. As originally written the chapter clearly established that anesthesiologists were the directors of the Anesthesia Care team and required that an anesthesiologist be Chief of the department. It came as no surprise, therefore, that the American Association of Nurse Anesthetists protested vigorously and threatened lawsuits. The Board of Commissioners became frightened and rescinded the statement that supervision had to be by an anesthesiologist and used the word "physician" instead. Although the change was somewhat of a disappointment, at least we had clearly established that anesthesiology was a clinical medical specialty in the eyes of JCAH and that a physician, not a technician, needed to be in overall supervision of the perioperative care of the patient.

During this time I was also appointed to head a task force to develop criteria for education of CRNAs. Many members of the ASA who conducted schools of nurse anesthesia felt that the quality of training in many of the hospital programs and, indeed, some of the university programs was totally inadequate. My task force working with representatives of AANA developed criteria for graduate training of CRNAs which included the eventual elimination of many unqualified programs. Our members argued that if CRNAs were going to be practicing as members of the anesthesia care team, anesthesiologists should have some input into the criteria for their education and certification.

In 1978 I was elected First Vice-President of the American Society of Anesthesiologists. I served as President-elect in 1979 through 1980 and as President from October, 1980 to October, 1981. The major focus during my years as an officer of ASA was quality of anesthesia care. Indeed, my address to the House of Delegates when I assumed the Presidency was entitled "Quality of Care: ASA's Raison d'Etre." Since my goal was improvement of quality of anesthesia care, I strongly supported the projects of the Peer Review Committee. My purpose was to exert peer pressure on the members of our society who were not practicing in accordance with the principles of ASA to improve the quality of anesthesia care. I believed then and continue to believe that it is incumbent upon our society to expose unethical and/or incompetent anesthesia practices.

During my year as President-elect I traveled to Bozeman, Montana to speak at the annual meeting of that society. Since the members were aware of my interest in quality of care, they suggested that ASA should have a program whereby the ASA could send representatives to review quality of care in various institutions throughout the country where there was not a sufficient number of anesthesiologists to perform peer review locally. I brought this proposal back to the Peer Review Committee and that stimulated the beginning of the "Onsite Review Program." It took some time to develop the program and it was Dr. Blancato who recommended the program to the House of Delegates. This program has served to terminate incompetent and unethical practices in a number of hospitals nationally.

In addition, I believed that the public had a right to know how to evaluate the quality of anesthesia care. It was obvious then, as it is today, that the public is ill-informed about what constitutes good quality anesthesia care. Accordingly, the ASA employed a public relations firm to (1) provide a course in speaker education so that we could provide a coherent message and (2) to provide access to media so that we could disseminate that message. Obviously, those who were providing high quality anesthesia care strongly supported this program. Conversely, those who were exploiting CRNAs and the public were not happy about the public becoming so well informed. Also some of the members of our society confused this program with an advertising or public relations program. It was never intended to be any sort of advertising program, but rather to educate the public to evaluate good quality anesthesia care and to insist upon it when entering a health care facility. We wanted people to know that the selection of an anesthesiologist was of equal importance to the selection of their surgeon or internist. I implemented this program during my year as President of ASA and, indeed, it was having an effect. The program continued during the presidency of Dr. Blancato. But this was a program that could not be completed in one or two years. Indeed, during the first two years, as would be expected, cost was rather high; but we anticipated that in the ensuing years the program could be maintained at much less cost. Unfortunately, the program was sharply curtailed before it could accomplish the goal that we hoped to attain. It is interesting that the membership of ASA is again requesting that a program of public education be instituted. It is certainly preferable for members of ASA to foster public education rather than leaving it to investigative television reporters who are frequently more interested in sensationalism than accuracy. In that regard, I recall the events surrounding the ABC 20/20 program that was presented in 1982. I was contacted by a representative of ABC's 20/20 program who said that they were interested in determining how anesthesia was practiced in a hospital setting. I was anxious to cooperate with what appeared to be a sincere attempt at public education. I guided the film crew through the entire perioperative course of a patient. Fortunately, the entire procedure went extremely well. They filmed the entire procedure and I assumed that they would show at least a substantial portion of the film to illustrate the importance of high quality anesthesia. Unfortunately, they misrepresented their purpose. Actually, they had some "horror story" material from other hospitals involving extremely poor quality anesthesia. Almost the entire program was devoted to exposing unethical and incompetent anesthesia care and less than 30 seconds to the successful anesthetic that was filmed at our hospital. With proper guidance we could have avoided this unfortunate incident.

Obviously, we did not learn the lesson very well because more recently ABC's "Day One" presented a similar program and again ASA's response was inadequate. The fact is that ASA should be proactive in exposing and expelling the unsavory members of our specialty who practice in a grossly unethical and incompetent manner. Further, we should educate the public about the quality of anesthesia care that they should demand. The emphasis on quality anesthesia care during my term of office was sustained by Dr. Pierce of Boston who initiated the very successful Patient Safety Program. These programs together with advances in technology have had a very beneficial effect in improving anesthesia care.

During my year as President of ASA I became involved in the exhibit for the Smithsonian Institute. This project had been under way for a number of years, but no real progress had been made. I appointed Dr. Leroy Vandam chairman of the Committee on Smithsonian Exhibit and was determined that we were going to get the exhibit displayed at the Smithsonian Institute. I, therefore, provided Dr. Vandam with the necessary administrative and financial support to accomplish this goal. Dr. Vandam and I made a special trip to Washington to visit the Curator at the museum. Dr. Vandam's eloquent presentation resulted in the acceptance of our exhibit on the "Management of Pain." We proudly presented this exhibit to the worldwide anesthesia community during the WFSA meeting held in Washington, D.C. in 1988. As President, I had appointed Dr. Jack Moyers of Iowa to Chair the Coordinating Committee for that meeting. He assembled a very dedicated team of anesthesiologists to serve on various subcommittees. I was appointed as Chair for Development and Publicity. We were able to raise approximately three quarters of a million dollars from various corporate donors in this country and abroad. In addition, we also obtained sponsorship for the various social functions that enhanced the meeting for our foreign visitors. The meeting was a huge success scientifically, financially, and socially. The WFSA was able to support many worthwhile programs with the money generated by this meeting. Dr. Jack Moyers, who served as Chair of the Coordinating Committee, deserves a great deal of credit for this accomplishment.

I believe that WFSA serves a very important function both in terms of developing brotherhood and understanding among people of the various countries and also in terms of providing medical help to many third world countries. During the meeting of the WSFA one of the things that I accomplished was bringing together the Japanese Society of Anesthesiology and the International Anesthesia Research Society (IARS). The first combined meeting was held in Japan and the second meeting was held under the auspices of IARS in Hawaii. The Japanese-American meetings were very successful and served to promote friendship and understanding among our colleagues.

In 1992 I was elected to the Committee on Representation to the American Medical Association. The other members of the committee were David Little, Pepper Jenkins, John Hattox, Richard Ament, Jess Weiss, and Jack Moyers. We devoted considerable time and effort to identifying and seeking solutions to the many problems faced by the medical community. Equally important, we worked to gain increased stature for our specialty. The AMA was very important in providing help for our legislative agenda and also in our interaction with the Joint Commission on Accreditation of Hospitals. As I pointed out previously, the AMA was very helpful in obtaining anesthesiology representation on the Professional and Technical Advisory Committee of the Joint Commission and also in getting the chapter on "Surgery and Anesthesia" adopted. The committee also worked with AMA to promote our mutual legislative agenda in Washington, D.C. There was great comradery among the members of the Committee on Representation and we worked together and socialized together very well. However, after a period of time, it became obvious that it was necessary for younger members to serve on the committee. Therefore, we adopted a system of term limits. There was a gradual change of committee personnel so that the newer members of the committee could become acquainted with the methodology used by the more experienced members to set forth our agenda. While a member of the Committee on Representation, I was appointed to serve on the Triple Committee (ASA, AMA, ABA) that nominated directors for the American Board of Anesthesiology. I had previously served in that capacity as a representative from ASA. During my tenure on the committee the representatives from ASA and AMA were able to terminate the practice of choosing directors by legacy, i.e., from the institution or vicinity of the retiring director. The process of selection became more democratic and provided a less parochial group. I believe that this change served to expand the vistas for new ideas with regard to the certification process and procedures.

In 1986, I was appointed to the Residency Review Committee for Anesthesiology. During my first year as a member of the committee I was elected vice-chair of the committee and two years later I was elected chair of the committee. During the six years that I served on the committee I believe that we accomplished a great deal. We made significant revisions in the "Special Requirements" and in addition, we were able to get "Pain Management" recognized as a subspecialty. Further, we worked on the concept of having unified accreditation for surgical, medical, and anesthesiology critical care. Although we were not able to accomplish this goal, the concept is very viable and I am convinced that it will come to fruition in the near future.

I have been privileged to serve my institution, my community, and the ASA in many capacities. My colleagues and others will have to determine what impact, if any, I may have made in my community and elsewhere. For myself, I am very proud of my former residents who practice in many hospitals in Michigan and other states, and I am proud of the department that I built in Detroit. No person makes good decisions all of the time, but I am convinced that my decision to enter the specialty of anesthesiology provided me with the most rewarding experiences that I could ever imagine.

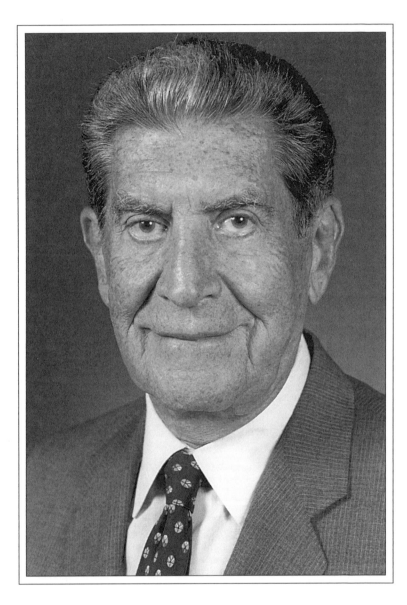

E.M. Papper, M.D., Ph.D.

19 October 1998

To Dr. Rima Matevosian
with all best wishes
E M Papper

THE PALATE
OF MY MIND

A Memoir

E.M. PAPPER, M.D., PH.D.

It is memory and not expectation
that gives unity and wholeness
to human existence.
— Hannah Arendt

PREFACE

At lunch, brown bag style, one day in March of 1996, Dr. George A. Silver and I were discussing some events in our lives that made a marked impression upon us. The story of his subtotal gastrectomy under emergency circumstances for hemorrhage is a tale which summarizes what surgery and anesthesia do to patients. Surgery is always dramatic. Anesthesia is always backstage.

If George had missed the anesthetic connection, it is certain most other people would also. George Silver is a brilliant physician who is one of the world's outstanding experts in Public Health and Social Medicine. He cares deeply about people and aspires to help create a better world where expert medical care will be available to all who need it. He is the retired Chairman of Yale's Department of Public Health. He has graciously permitted me to tell his story.

Scheduled as an emergency for subtotal gastrectomy to stop the bleeding from an artery in the duodenum, on Thanksgiving Day of 1954, Dr. Mark Ravitch was asked to perform the operation. Silver was the head of the Social Medicine program at Montefiore Hospital in New York City and Ravitch, the Chief of Surgery at Mt. Sinai in New York. Elliott Hurwitt, Montefiore's Surgeon-in-Chief was away on vacation. Ravitch and Silver were neighbors and friends. The name of the anesthesiologist is unknown. This blank spot illustrates the problem. The surgeon has a high profile and even so discerning a person as George Silver does not recall the name of his anesthesiologist.

George was delighted with the results of his operation. He told me:

"The surgery was so good that I was out of bed on the first post operative day. I had a soft diet on the second post operative day and was home in a week. On the tenth day, Mitzi (his wife) and I were in Jamaica on vacation. I was back to work shortly thereafter."

I then said to him:

"George, that is a splendid recovery and your surgery was performed very well by Mark Ravitch. But I think your attribution of how you progressed so fast, especially getting to Jamaica so quickly was wrong. Dr. X, the unknown anesthesiologist, got you there. He took care of all the rest of George Silver except the control of the duodenal hemorrhage during the procedure. He even took care of the *consequences* of that hemorrhage."

George smiled and said:

"Why don't you tell that story in your Memoir? Everyone can identify with me, the patient. Your continually making the point of the unappreciated role of the anesthesiologist will be overcome."

And so I tell all of you a story of real events, often misunderstood.

"George, I thank you for the permission to tell your story. I know that Dr. X would also appreciate your agreement that *he* sent you to Jamaica if he knew about you now!!"

Backstage makes possible what goes in the front of the stage.

INTRODUCTION

This book is my story. It is designed to explore, describe and analyze with comment on my life, particularly, my contributions to my specialty in medicine of anesthesiology. I was, in many respects, fortunate to have been part of the "Joshua" generation, following the "Moses" role of Waters, Rovenstine, Lundy, McMechan, Wood and several others. Second generation pioneers live a heady life. They have to understand and deal with some opinions differing from those of their elders and upon them falls the duty of widening and popularizing the new "religion." In the vast majority of instances, there was substantial agreement with their mentors who were the real pioneers. They (or we) had a grave responsibility and a very gaudy opportunity to do very much good for patients and for the development of education for physicians and patients, based upon sound fundamental science. Not everyone enjoys the challenge of doing something important and worthwhile. The possibility of failure, which is real, never entered my mind (nor my spirit). It was go for broke. Bring the message to the medical community, for *their* benefit and the benefit of *their* patients. How could one lose if the material was good, the mission generous for others and the process exciting and delightful. I felt lucky to be "chosen" by the fates for a role that would keep me on my toes and would always give me the feeling of giving, not receiving.

I suppose I did receive. Honors and respect developed in due course. Reward had to be the satisfaction of improving the public health of a nation, by helping to make its anesthetic care safe, then respectable and finally, outstanding. The privilege of discovery, often called research, and the careful development of leaders in anesthesiology were terrestrial rewards for all of us that exceeded the unknown potential of celestial benevolence. Life was enthusiastically worth living. Not too many of us have a chance to contribute to a society in need. I did, and I am grateful for the opportunity.

How should these events be described? It is an epic, and I could start "in media res." It is also a straightforward story, with a beginning, a middle and an end. I believe it best to start at the beginning. Most of my friends and most anesthesiologists think that the second wave of pioneers was born as adults, lived a short comet speed life, and disappeared in middle age. I think it useful for the reader to know that the "pre-contribution" to anesthesiology years had a marked influence in developing the person in whom they had (or have) an interest. I also believe it is important to learn something about the life of a pioneer after his/her period of maximum influence and activity is gone. Will this knowledge help cast light in how we, in anesthesiology, can build a tradition? If so, will it help the self-esteem and perhaps inspire somewhat the spirit of all anesthesiologists in these dark and daunting times?

I then decided (with the approval of the Wood Library-Museum Committee who invited me to write this book) to write a memoir of these events rather than an autobiography. A memoir consists of the description of thoughts, events and activities as I remember them. In contrast, an autobiography is a form of history and requires documentation and a different level of objectivity in contrast to subjective remembrances. The spirit of the descriptions ought to be lighter and perhaps more controversial. A comment on this approach is found in the statement of the 18th Century sage, Samuel Johnson, who wrote in the Rambler: "I have often thought that there has rarely passed a life of which a judicial and faithful narrative would not be useful" (Samuel Johnson, Rambler 60, Saturday, 13 October, 1750). This comment is ample support to tell my story my way.

The question arose as to what should one tell in a memoir. What, in short, is of interest and what may be of importance to a reader, presumably an anesthesiologist, although possibly other types of physicians and maybe even some non-medical people would want to know about these experiences? Do they share the attitudes that I possess, the most important of which is the fact that one can not really understand a special field in medicine and for that matter, most other forms of human endeavor without knowing what else was going at the time in other areas of human culture? Does my work need the explanation of understanding me, my childhood and my subsequent growth? How much is needed? How much is good? Probably the knowledge of what makes a person and what he becomes is of importance in understanding why his views are what they are as they develop.

Then there are all the unknown factors of serendipity. Chance events have a major impact on the course of education, development and personality that any individual, myself obviously included, experiences. The environment in which growing up took place; education and its impacts and the nature of significant economic factors within the family have an influence on thoughts and actions. Certainly the wide and important influence of societal forces also affects growth and development. Whether opportunities were seized or not is important. Unconscious forces may be crucial to the evolution of an individual and are individualistically variable. Therefore, in the spirit of these observations, I have decided to describe some of my early childhood and early development. These events may contribute to understanding my activities better in later years. Is the child the "father of the man" as Wordsworth sings? I think he is.

I wish to acknowledge the intelligence, the skilled use of a word processor and the vast and important help in producing this book, of Mr. Lawrence Soto, without whose work it could not have been written.

THE PALATE OF MY MIND
CHILDHOOD

I was born in New York City on Manhattan island in the district known then, as it is now, as Harlem on the 12th of July, 1915. So unimportant was my birth to the young doctor who attended my mother, Lillian Weitzner Papper and my father Max Papper, that I wasn't recorded in the official annals of New York City as of that date. My birth certificate has always been eight days wrong by being recorded as the 20th of July, 1915. This is better than some friends who are contemporaneous in which the birth certificate simply read baby boy or baby girl. One must be satisfied therefore with some advance over total anonymity.

This error caused no great harm, except when my eighteenth birthday was at hand. My father was a very generous supporter of my brother and me in many ways, mostly by giving of himself, since we were of lower middle class origins and there was very little money available. He taught me to drive an automobile when I was about thirteen. I drove under carefully controlled conditions in places where it would not expose me or other drivers to any danger. These might have been short vacations in the Castskill borscht circuit during a few days in the summer and the likes of that experience. However, such is youth! When I wanted to take my driving test at the age of eighteen and applied to do so on the 12th of July, 1933, I was told with no great courtesy by the authorities of the Bureau of Motor Vehicles that I was not eligible for a license even if I should pass the driving test until the 20th of July because that was my official birthday.

An eight day change seems trivial now, even to me, but at the time it carried with it a force of great destructive power. I was very upset at being deprived, by the trappings of legality, of having the precious driving license I yearned to possess. It also taught me one of the lessons that I should have learned earlier. Inaccuracies inevitably lead to difficulty if they happen to come into conflict with aspirations that must cope with such a possibility. I also had driven into me the clear lesson that one should be very certain of the facts and the data before embarking on any activity of importance to oneself or to others affected by it.

We lived in Harlem for about a year and a half and whether I should, from the standpoint of the unconscious qualities of the newborn infant, have any recollections of this period I have never been able to determine. The fact is that I have no memories of it and yet always enjoyed two aspects of the experience. My mother, presumably to stake out an aura of respectability, always told me that Harlem at the time of my birth was a very pleasant suburb of New York inhabited by fairly recent immigrants to the United States, most of whom were of Italian, Irish and Jewish ancestry.

Both of my parents emigrated to New York City but from different parts of the pre World War I Austro-Hungarian Empire. My mother arrived at the tender age of three or four and my father, when he was approaching the age where conscription into the armed forces of Austria-Hungary was possible, emigrated in order to avoid a military draft. The leaving of the "old country" with its oppressions to Jews, its obsession with nationalistic grandeur at the turn of the 20th Century leading to the catastrophic events of war, brutality and misery that the 20th Century acquired from these apparently excessively grandiose feelings — these were common causes for the emigration of young men. The women who came presumably did so because of parents or occasionally, as was partially true with my mother, the death of a parent and the need to be with someone who could take care of a young child whose father had died in her very early childhood.

My parents desired to be nearer to their family and also to be in a more settled and more identifiably populated Jewish neighborhood. They moved to what was then known as the Lower East Side in Manhattan and is now part of Greenwich Village East. The Lower East Side of my very early childhood was densely populated by Jewish settlers, most of whom were observant in their classical religious orthodoxy of the European Shtetl. There were, of course, also in that part of Manhattan island a small and increasingly strident Jewish population who were radical politically and who enjoyed the first successes of the Bolshevik Revolution which took place in 1917 in the formation of the Soviet Union as a reaction to the Czarist oppression of Imperial Russia and which also took the country out of World War I. This fascinating but strange mix of orthodox Jews and very secular leftist and radical Jews I remember with vivid recall.

My orthodoxy at that period was unimpaired but my interest and fascination with the secular radical Jews was also a very remarkable part of my experience. There was hope for a better future in America for both groups.

My maternal grandmother lived with us and she was much more familiar to me than my father's mother. She was a pretty tough lady who had to be tough to have survived her youthful widowhood in Europe with all of the sociological disabilities that any widow had. Judgments about marital status were hostile to many young widows. In America, she was able to work and earn enough money before the turn of the century to bring her three children who were living with relatives in Europe, since their father was dead, to this country. She did a magnificent job under the kind of pressures that would be excessive stress to many people in today's world.

One wonders, in admiration, whether the fact that a person had no viable option over a hundred years ago was an adequate stimulus to just getting the job done. Was this behavior healthier or a problem that would impede the evolution and growing toward Americanization which was the goal of my family? I am still stunned with approval at the courage, the hard and focused work that these new immigrants produced and the sense of value and ethics that they developed in their offspring. Not everybody was wonderful by a long way, but it is astonishing to remember how many of these Jewish immigrants lived by what is commonly, and in my view mistakenly, identified as the Protestant ethic in the United States. This ethic goes back much further in time. It had its origins in poverty or near poverty and the realization of its victims that there was no option but to do the job and hope that the American dream was not one of illusion. If you worked hard and honestly you could "make it."

All was not wine and roses with my maternal grandmother. She lived with us because my mother, her only daughter, felt that it was the responsibility of a *female* descendant to look after an aging parent. Grandma, called Baba, was still in her fifties, but she was "retired"!

Thus were sown the seeds of trouble in our household. Although I was more or less exempt from the daily mischief since I was her eldest grandchild, I could see that she seemed to be the focus, if not the cause of intense trouble between my parents.

Baba did not contribute to the economy nor the work load of our household. She viewed herself as retired and exempt from any contribution to us and became self absorbed to an advanced degree. She refused even to baby-sit for me and my brother despite her alleged love and devotion to us. My parents were reduced to taking us with them if they wanted to go anywhere. There obviously were no servants and paid baby sitters were not affordable. The result was some mayhem for me. We were taken to inexpensive poker games on Saturday nights. At midnight or later, after a couple of hours of sleep, we were awakened and taken home. My brother and I never played cards later in life. It was total rejection pushed by an unpleasant experience. Of course, Baba was blamed for not "sitting" with us.

Furthermore, she was very unpleasant to my father, which was hard to do. He was always very accommodating, especially to my mother. She breathed a wish and he hastened to comply — except about her mother. The events reached epic proportions. Pop and Baba did not speak to each other nor acknowledge each other's presence until her death in 1949. Ironically and sadly, he outlived her only a little over a year. Such is conflict *inside* the four walls. What did Baba do during all her "free" hours? She played cards and occasionally went to the synagogue *if* she liked the Rabbi. In all fairness to my father's viewpoints of her, Baba's daughters-in-law were sympathetic to *him*, but would have no part of having her live with them.

My father's story was a different one and somewhat difficult for me to envision. He was born in Austria-Hungary and raised by his paternal grandfather who owned a large farm, replete with horses and even servants. It was hard for me to imagine that any of the Jews of the Austro-Hungarian Empire could have been so well off. But Pop always maintained that his grandfather was wealthy He did not know his mother who left for the United States when he was a small child. He never forgave her for abandoning him. His father had died when he was little in a accident that involved horses, the details unknown to me. It was very difficult for me to see his elegant life in a Jewish family who must have shared in the difficulties of the age. Yet years later when we moved to Brooklyn to be in what he always called the country and to see him ride on the bridle path of Ocean Parkway, near Prospect Park, in a gorgeous riding outfit (where he found or bought it was a secret) with English saddle and ride like a dream, I knew he could not have acquired this skill without the experience that he himself always described in the old country. In trying to unravel the geographical aspects and their possible impacts on my parents, I became convinced that the part of Austria-Hungary that both families came from was really in a piece of Poland that is known as Galicia and was moved around like a pawn among the then great powers of Central and Eastern Europe, i.e., Imperial Russia, Prussia and Austria-Hungary's Empire. This is the only geographical solution that makes any sense to me.

I had always imagined the locus of the living places for central and eastern European Jews as being poverty stricken, slum like houses with the possible exception of the schools that taught religion, Torah, Talmud and Midrash and the synagogue that they supported. These were literally examples of cleanliness next to godliness. All of my mental images of my family's places of origin were incomplete and largely erroneous. When I learned more about these matters, my admiration for their courage in emigrating to gain spiritual, intellectual and physical relief from oppression of the mind and cruelty and violence to the body that they suffered in Europe in our century of violence was greatly increased.

After about two years of living in the Lower East side of Manhattan my parents chose to move to Brooklyn where they felt they were going to be in the country. The first move in that direction certainly didn't accomplish their purpose since financially they couldn't afford it. They lived in an apartment house that was very simple, but clean and undoubtedly all that they could afford. The neighborhood had more than its fair share of violence.

I was the eldest of the grandchildren and at this particular time, the only grandchild. I remember a happy early childhood despite the nearly slum like nature of the area with its attendant violence of street gangs in a neighborhood of mixed backgrounds and hostilities. There was a mixture of people of Irish descent, Italian stock and Jews from central and eastern Europe. We lived near the Brooklyn Jewish Hospital. There were all too many instances of young people, especially young boys, being taken there for the treatment of knife, blackjack and occasionally gunshot wounds due to the street warfare.

However my childhood experiences of this period when I was four, five or six were quite happy despite the street violence. My mother often took me to nearby Prospect Park to visit the beautiful Japanese gardens there. This environment was pleasant, quiet and bucolic in its simplicity and its peacefulness. It was almost as though we were lifted out of a congested world of strife and violence into the anteroom of a glorious and peaceful Heaven. I also had a wonderful time playing in my aunt Pauline's home because she doted on me as the only child of the extended family. Her first child, my cousin Walter, was not yet born. He arrived when I was five years old. I therefore had all the attention one could possibly have from a solicitous and loving mother and also the attentions of love and affection from a very maternal nurturing person, my aunt Pauline. It was her Romanian origins that first introduced me to foods like eggplant and polenta with its various synonyms. She called it mamaliga. It was only later that I learned these other names for the wonderful peasant dish made from yellow corn meal or maize.

I don't recall particularly any playing of games although I enjoyed, with very great pleasure, being the only child among a family of adults. It was particularly important to have that kind of family structure for children because at that time the men of the family worked incredibly hard and were seldom home when I was awake. It was not yet the time for women to be in the workplace. The men worked for very modest incomes despite the long hours. The small business of my two uncles and my father slowly improved over time but they never were even close to being financially comfortable until the period after World War II.

Eventually, these arrangements no longer suited my parents and my uncles and they all moved further out to areas in Brooklyn that could be reasonably considered as the "country," by their standards. We moved to an area in Flatbush in Brooklyn that was approximately midway between Coney Island and the Atlantic Ocean on one side and Prospect Park and the then beautiful section of Brooklyn on the other. Our street was unpaved and people owned domestic animals like goats and sheep as well as pets like dogs and cats. Ostensibly we moved because of my mother's pregnancy with my brother, but I think it was time for them to be in a neighborhood where they could really enjoy what they must have imagined the real America to be like. They bought a very modest home; a semi-detached single family house in Flatbush. In 1922, shortly after our move, my brother was born and it was a delightful event in our family. Everybody was extraordinarily happy to have this new infant in the family.

HIGH SCHOOL

In 1928 I entered Boys High School, also in Brooklyn. The high school had an enormously strong reputation in academic strength; it had only males; and it was difficult to gain admission. All of which seemed to appeal both to me and to my parents.

Boys High School was in many ways a wonderful adventure and an agreeable learning process. Its strong academic reputation caused a meeting in the school's auditorium at which the principal, Dr. Eugene Colligan, addressed the entire student population of which I was a newly arrived member and castigated all of the boys. In his view, Boys High School's academic achievements had fallen on hard times. For the first time in many years Boys High School *alone* did not succeed in acquiring a majority of the total number of New York State Regents' Scholarships given to *all* the other public high schools in New York City combined.

Learning in a very traditional mode was a pleasure in that it caused no serious disturbance of equanimity. Rarely was there an innovative and adventurous teacher in that system. In most instances the assignments were routine and depended more on memory than creative thought. This was the pattern for that period in public education at the high school level. The teachers were wonderful and thought of themselves as elite. The students were typically lower middle class and they even had a good football team despite their academic excellence. I remember vividly a football hero called Rudy Cohen who was a fine student in addition to being a massive effective lineman on the team. The students with strong academic records seemed to be very much enamored of this type of athleticism. There were other notable experiences at Boys High, particularly with two teachers who were of major importance to me.

In this period between the two World Wars it seemed a little odd to many of my friends that I should enjoy taking as many German courses as were available. It is not that the choices were exceedingly large. One had a choice of Latin, German, French and I think Spanish as options and had to take two of these languages in order to graduate and be eligible for college.

German was taught by Mr. Otto Beckert and a wonderful teacher he was. Any student who could pronounce a diphthong or a word with an umlaut nearly correctly was almost heroic in his eyes. He was a sweet, gentle and highly competent educator in the language and culture that he obviously loved. Despite the anti-German feelings of that particular period, a small number of students, including me, very much enjoyed our experience in both the German language and the German culture provided by Mr. Beckert. The only defect that I could see in retrospect was the fact that much reading, some writing and very little speaking was part of the way that a language different from English was taught. I could read the words with a reasonable accent but speaking was an impossibility or at least a very severe burden and was not encouraged either by him or by other teachers of foreign languages. This defect of American views towards foreign languages worsened with time until probably well after World War II when it became important to understand that one had to be able to speak the language as well as to read it or hear it. However with all of these criticisms, Mr. Beckert remained a favorite teacher and I can almost visualize him sixty-odd years later still striding up and down the aisles of the classroom between the rows of seats and responding with flagrant joy at the efforts that students were making to please him as well as to learn German.

My other hero at this time was Mr. Michael Vessa, a teacher of classical languages and culture. Latin was his great love and I think sometimes because of his Italian ancestry, he assumed straight and pure descent from the ancient classic Romans. Michael Vessa read Latin aloud like an ancient Roman. The "dead" language was very much alive as it emerged from his larynx. We were studying Cicero and one could almost visualize the great poet as the classical phrases assumed life mediated by sound. It was wonderful. Occasionally, as the spirit seized him, Mr. Vessa *spoke* Latin to us, but did not insist in our doing so. Perhaps he thought our barbaric tongues would mutilate his beloved language. It was Mr. Vessa who became a very important part of my life when I reached the last semester of the last year and was about to graduate.

As graduation day approached, I had the misfortune of being felled by an attack of rubella (German measles). It definitely is not an amusing experience. On my recovery, I was well enough to take the Regents Examinations and won a scholarship of one hundred dollars per year for four years. I was also chosen Valedictorian and made a speech that will not survive as immortal. I won four medals, including a surprise award in American History from the Daughters of the American Revolution, a group not exactly noted for their liberal qualities.

COLUMBIA COLLEGE

Mr. Vessa deemed me worthy of being given the opportunity for a splendid education on the collegiate level. However we were in the grip of the Great Depression. My family had very little money to spare beyond the essentials of the sort of living I have described. Michael Vessa was an alumnus of Columbia College and I believe also of the graduate school. Fortunately for me, he was also the advisor for students concerning college admission.

In the early thirties it wasn't so much a question of which campus to visit with my parents or where I wanted to go to college, or what plans there would be for social partying or other lovely leisurely activities. The issue for a New York youngster with some academic talent was to go to the City College of New York which was an exceptionally splendid institution of free tuition or to seek admission to Columbia College provided one could get a scholarship or a work opportunity or both to pay the very modest tuition at Columbia in those days. Going to college somewhere other than New York City, was financially impossible for most people in the economic circumstances of my family. Vessa was convinced that I deserved to go Columbia (a view that I have cherished the rest of my life since it brought so much good to me). He arranged a supplement of my Regent's Scholarship, which was $100.00 per year, by getting the rest of my tuition supported by Columbia. I also had the opportunity of delivering newspapers to faculty members prior to starting my own classes and earned some money doing so.

The time of the Depression was extremely onerous for families and students who had academic abilities because so many were deprived of opportunities for higher education for economic reasons. Therefore I viewed myself as exceptionally fortunate to be sponsored by Mr. Vessa at Columbia and to gain admission as a Freshman in 1931.

The environment of Morningside Heights was, at first, a very large and somewhat confusing one to me. Ours was one of the smaller sized classes in Columbia's 20th Century experience, largely due to the economic impact of the Depression. Vastly different is today's experience on Morningside Heights in New York when almost all of the students are residential and for the last fifteen years or so, women have been admitted to the all male College of my day. In 1931 I suppose some 75 or 80 percent of the students did not live on the campus because they couldn't afford to and there weren't enough dormitory facilities in any event. I was one of the commuters and had to spend a large amount of time (three hours daily) going in both directions on the subway. The cost was five cents each way — in contrast to the one dollar and twenty five cents which it is in 1996.

However aside from the fact that I had little campus life, I found the experience at Columbia to be exhilarating beyond belief. Here I was, a youth of sixteen raised contentedly and happily in the provincial and very small world of a lower middle class son of Jewish European immigrants, and found myself in a world swirling with intellectual strength and with marvelous exposure to many different ideas which I knew nothing about prior to beginning as a student at Columbia. I couldn't wait to grasp one learning opportunity after another and one of the things that Mr. Vessa advised me to do was to try to take more advanced courses than freshmen usually were allowed by taking examination for advanced placement. I succeeded in doing this in English and Mathematics, in German and History. However fortunately for me, the great course now seventy-five years old known as Contemporary Civilization was required of all freshmen and sophomores. Without this vital course, the exposure of young men to the miracles of Western Civilization (with all of its dead white males) would not have occurred. Most students are not as competent as a great faculty in knowing what is good for them! It was also a time when the leading scholars of a famous university were happy to teach undergraduates, possibly because they really liked it and possibly also because the economy suffered from twenty percent unemployment. Unemployment possibilities for faculty members must have been stimuli to even a gifted group of educators to work at teaching. Classes were small and teaching by graduate students was unknown. We learned quickly how really exceptional the faculty was and how very able they were in dealing with young uneducated and unformed boys about to become young men.

It was in these exhilarating days that I heard about the breakage of much intellectual crockery by Mortimer Adler, recently departed from Columbia, who became a very close and cherished friend years later. Our affection for Columbia was a knitting force between us. It was there also that I first met the distinguished historian, Professor Jacques Barzun, who was then a newly minted assistant professor of History. He was about to burst upon the intellectual scene because of his great intellect, great elegance and particular interest in young people who were aspiring to the things that he thought were important. My close relationship with him has lasted for a long time and I view Jacques Barzun as one of my great heroes. I feel most fortunate in having had the pleasure of his friendship into the ninth decade of my life and toward the end of that decade of his. There were Nobel Laureates, Pulitzer Prize winners who taught us in classes as small as eight to ten. Occasionally a lecture course might have as many as forty students. In fact, almost everyone seemed to view himself as fortunate to be there although there was a radical Marxist movement at Columbia as there was elsewhere in the country.

The pro-Communist activities were understandable because of the results of the severe Depression. Some students were expelled for radical activities, but leftist politics became more or less acceptable as Franklin Roosevelt and his New Deal were appearing on the now closer horizon.

My entry into college at Columbia at the age of sixteen brought an unexpected and painful conflict despite the other wonderful experiences. It was fortunate in retrospect that it occurred in an environment as powerful intellectually as Columbia. The problem, for me, was one of searching for stability in a wildly exciting but chaotic universe. Perhaps a few words of explanation of the provincial nature of a young lad of sixteen brought up in the tight security of an Orthodox Jewish education is needed. The only real departure from approved ritual observation in my life was the occasional movie that we saw on Friday nights. Travel and the handling of money — both forbidden — were required. I always felt an uneasy sensation of sin, but more or less accommodated to my parents' desire to go to the movies. It was a transient period of release to them from the hard work of the week. But it left a negative feeling in me and a hostility to the movies that has lasted. There were questions to which I could not find appropriate answers. The sacred five books, the Talmud or the Mishna did not provide solutions for me. Family life was also both narrow and comfortable in the sense that all the people I knew were in similar classless distinctions of marginal financial support which was always generated by a working father.

The explosive nature of the much larger world of Morningside Heights and its very great brain power together with the incredibly open and advanced cultural course work to which I was exposed were exciting and yet very upsetting emotionally and intellectually. All of these experiences produced many areas of challenge and uncertainty in my previous very comfortable life in Brooklyn, New York as an Orthodox observant Jew. I had only once crossed west of the Hudson River beyond New Jersey and that was to go to Philadelphia. I had never been in any Christian church nor had I tasted non-kosher food.

The nature of the conflict of religions illustrated by events such as the Crusades, the Ghetto life of Jews throughout the many centuries in the Diaspora after the fall of Jerusalem and the destruction of the first and then the second temples and the long time faceless hatreds of anti-Semitism were disturbing to experience in my reading. All of these made a major impact on my young and naive mind. I felt suddenly cast adrift upon a sea of a new adventure which was tremendously unsettling while at the same time it was forcing liberation of a mind.

All this was associated with the massive hit of the Great Depression which had begun in October of 1929. One of my college classmates said that our arrival on Morningside Heights as freshmen students in 1931 was celebrated by the closing of the banks. A very wry and ironic statement. Our family had no money in any bank and it didn't really make any difference whether the banks were open or closed from our standpoint. However I knew enough to understand that this event was depicting an American failure of such magnitude that suicides and wide and devastating suffering were unfortunately commonplace. The ability of my young and inexperienced mind to grasp all the implications of these burdensome events was grossly inadequate.

The natural first effort for me to cope with these problems was to go back to the safe environment of the local synagogue and talk over the new challenges and problems with the Rabbi and some of my favorite teachers, especially Mr. Michael Vessa, my beloved Latin teacher at Boys High School. These discussions seemed [to be] disappointingly ineffective in helping me think through my dilemmas. The Rabbi was, if anything, somewhat angry with me for my new feelings of doubt and questioning of our religion. He likened me to a young Jew in classical Greece who elected to try to become a Greek "so that he could be like all the others." I had neither courage nor knowledge to challenge that discussion further. I felt letdown. It was my first encounter with adults whom I liked and respected who could not understand the violent upheavals and turbulence precipitated by the insecurities of belief. The hostile opposing cultures to my own, as I saw the problem, left me terribly confused.

I left these discussions with more doubt and discontent and started to talk about them with such people as Professor Irwin Edman who had befriended me. His friendship was very fortunate for me. Edman was Professor of Philosophy at Columbia and he clearly understood the nature of my conflicts much better than I did. Professor Edman suggested talking with some of the counseling people on the campus including the Jewish Chaplain and also the Catholic Chaplain, Father George Ford. He thought these men would understand very well the problems I was pursuing and would be able to help in their resolution. I elected to see Father Ford of whom my Catholic student friends were extremely fond.

Almost intuitively I recognized that more knowledge about the Catholic church, at least as Father Ford interpreted it, would be useful for me and we arranged to have several sessions. I asked him to treat those sessions in a more serious way than simply counseling. I thought that I might be attracted to the Roman Catholic Church because it seemed to have appropriate answers for most of the serious questions that were going on in my mind. Ironically, I think as I viewed it in retrospect later on,

I was seeking the same kind of stability that Orthodox Judaism had had for me and was no longer possible to accept. I mistakenly thought that the Catholic solution to religious convictions might be better for me. Obviously this was an enormously radical and dangerous idea for me to express to my family or to even my friends. Therefore, I asked Father Ford to work with me and to give me instruction in the Catholic church because I wanted to know whether it was where I belonged. Could it solve the doubts that were ravaging my comfort level and should I seriously consider conversion to the Catholic church? He was very kind and as one of my Catholic friends who was devoted to him remarked he was so good (and dangerous?) that the Church never even made him a Monsignor! We worked together about once a week for several months and my doubts increased in some respects. I began to understand that conversion was not a possible solution for my confusion. I learned a great deal about the Church, its history, its strengths, its miscues, its catastrophic Inquisition in the late Middle Ages and early Renaissance; and its anti-Semitism. In short I got a great education. However I think that I was waiting for Father Ford's interpretation of all of these apparently disconnected ramblings. My suffering from a severe spiritual angst was not greatly abated despite the warmth of his friendship.

During one of these sessions I asked straight out whether I would feel better and whether things would be better if I were baptized and decided to convert. Much to my amazement and relief combined, he suggested to me that he thought I should not be converted to the Church because I really did not have any conviction that transfer of religion to Christianity from Judaism would provide the personal comfort level I was seeking. I simply did not have the faith that was required. Converted or not, my troubles had to be worked out in some other way. Other means had to be sought to find a way through the spiritual and intellectual uncertainties and difficulties I was experiencing. Father Ford suggested that, in his view, the attractions of the Catholic church to me were its pageantry, its glorious music (to which I am still very devoted) and to the humanistic interest in fine art that were the results of the taste and interests of the various Popes, Cardinals and Bishops over the many centuries. I didn't realize until many years later that the love of Christian art that I experienced also had a down side to it. The various artists over the centuries, especially at the time when the Church was dominant in Europe, were not free to paint whatever they liked and while it is not necessarily true that the artists were irreligious, it was much easier for them to pursue the paintings of events and principals in the Bible of both the Old and New Testaments but especially those of the Christian gospels. The subject matter, therefore, had to be acceptable to the Church and it took a long time before I understood how that happened. I began to realize that I would have to find my way myself whether or not I chose to remain a Jew or to become a Christian.

The issue was settled not too long thereafter. There was a sterling example in my immediate environment of reasons for conversion. Thomas Merton was several classes ahead of me and while I didn't know him well, I knew about him. He started as a Protestant and not only became a Catholic but became a priest, then a monk with the most severe restrictions on daily living. He was to become a Trappist monk and accepted a vow of silence. He, of course, became a very important figure in the Church as well as a great literary artist. The interpretation and lesson I drew [from all these experiences] was that while the problems may have been the same or, if not the same, similar in nature for young people who were pried loose from their comfortable childhood environments and [therefore] restricted experiences, the solutions were as variable as the people and their instinctual behaviors demanded. I think I learned what I believe the contemporary civilization course was trying to teach. Varied interpretations of the past and of the present were not only permissible but were encouraged as long as they included tolerance for differences from others and respect for intellectual dissent from an orthodoxy of any kind.

This thought sounds as though an optimal environment could be found, but imperfections in human behavior were always going to disturb in some way the equanimity that could be derived from such thinking. For example, only ten percent of my class or less were Jewish. There were no blacks. There were no women, which I now believe was an unconscious discrimination but didn't even think about at the time. There were fraternities that were hallmarks of homogeneity. They discriminated against all students who were not homogeneous white Protestant males. Jewish fraternities existed, but seemed out of place. There were secret societies at the College which had Indian sounding names (now they would be called Native American, of course) and they were not open to anyone but the non-Indian ruling majority white Anglo-Saxon Protestant males.

The sorting out of some of these matters lessened my tensions to a reasonable degree and made it possible to concentrate on the vast educational opportunities which this great College at that important time in my life permitted. I believe that whatever contributions I was able to make in my life's work were made possible and greatly enhanced by my Columbia education. I could thrive because the wonderful new experiences outweighed the dead hand of bigotry.

In my undergraduate student days at Columbia there was a system insuring the satisfactory development from basic courses to more demanding advanced courses. The system was operated by giving "maturity credits," as they were called, for advanced courses. A certain number of "maturity credits" which guaranteed the student's progress from simple to more advanced courses had to be achieved for graduation. This arrangement, from my point of view, gave flexibility and opportunity to take advanced courses in several fields and not be confined to one field such as foreign language or biology.

There were also very interesting advanced courses that required faculty approval to enter. One very important one was known as Colloquium, was one of these. Admission was granted to a student only in the junior or senior year by the faculty conducting the course. The course consisted of original important literary works and discussion was seminar in type. This was as near a graduate program as an undergraduate college could have. Great stress was placed by the faculty upon the reading of original material.

This system produced in some of us a rather interesting and exciting development. If one could achieve taking advanced courses as well as the wonderful one contemporary civilization, which was required, it became feasible to develop skills in more than one field and often several fields. I was fortunate enough to take advantage of this arrangement and was able to achieve some skill in English Literature, History, Biological Sciences and Chemistry to the point where I could qualify as a pre-science person for Graduate or Professional School and at the same time also qualify for advanced graduate work in the Humanities. This presentation of intellectual riches at Columbia was the source of very great pleasure despite the need for serious concentration. These needs and capabilities required both talent and hard work.

Because of the impact of the Great Depression some of these avenues seemed like obstacles rather than highways to performance. In order to pursue any one of these paths further I would need a scholarship or fellowship support depending on which route was selected. At the time, I thought of pursuing a career in academic philosophy. I have often wondered how I would have turned out had I pursued that career. Chance and opportunity may arrive in many guises. I would not have had a medical career in Anesthesiology if I had secured a fellowship in Philosophy in the mid 1930s and therefore would have missed the many wonderful experiences that I had. Were there other events that I did miss because of the choice I made? I will never know!

MEDICAL SCHOOL

Professor Edman suggested to me that I do something in one of the sciences where it might have been possible to get either fellowship or graduate student support and then return to

Philosophy when things were looser and more feasible in the world of the Humanities. He had suggested Engineering and my view was that Engineering would not be good for me. In the 1930s, the engineers that I knew were building bridges or sewers. These activities were of no interest whatsoever to me. He thought that Medicine might be a useful substitute since it had elements of the blending of the Humanities with Life Sciences.

The same problem about scholarship help occurred for medical school and there were no student loans of the sort that are available today. Although as an offsetting consideration, tuition was considerably more manageable than it is today.

By a combination of scholarship help, family assistance and securing various part time jobs, it was possible to negotiate this settlement if I could qualify for admission to a medical school. I made three applications. The first application was to the College of Physicians and Surgeons at Columbia. I was granted an interview and at the age of nineteen was thought by the Admissions Committee to be too young to enter medical school with its problems of dealing with human illness, death and disease. I was advised to stay another year or perhaps even two for the purpose of maturing. This was not feasible for me for financial reasons. There was no way I could afford to wait for the development of maturity even if I agreed with the Admissions Committee's assessment.

My application to Cornell, despite being second in my class at Columbia, was not even answered, a situation which I have never understood except that there were quotas against minority students. New York University was a more comfortable situation, at least at the entry point, in that there appeared to be either minimal or no discrimination against Jews, Italians, Irish or other minorities [and they were known as the producer of practicing physicians for the city of New York, which was a healthy thing to do.] Their teaching hospital was the famous Bellevue Hospital where learning was a wonderful experience. New York University was also willing to help with assistance in job support and also a partial scholarship toward tuition payments. Not being able to afford to wait and seeing its strong and sturdy reputation as a major educator of New York physicians, I elected to go to New York University.

When I told Professor Edman of my decision he thought this plan was fine and I began medical school in the fall of 1934. Toward the end of the first year in medical school, Professor Edman indicated that a fellowship in Philosophy might be forthcoming if I was ready to come back to the Columbia campus.

The first year was very difficult although a very attractive and interesting one. I elected to stay another year and found the second year even more interesting in substance and content despite the unpleasant environment of some faculty members continuing to be unreasonably rough on students. When Professor Edman once again suggested that it was time to "return" I had a difficult decision to make. I decided to stay in medical school and confer with him and perhaps other of my friends at Morningside Heights periodically. I decided that I wanted to finish the course in medical school. My enjoyment of the content of medical education was always great. When I was invited to do research in the Department of Medicine in the Metabolic and Endocrine Laboratories of Dr. Elaine Ralli, I was delighted to do so. It required an additional accommodation to find the time to be a student and a researcher who was attached to one of the more senior people in her division. I learned a great deal from her and from her colleagues while doing research as a student in both third and fourth years. I was so interested in the elements of research related to diabetes and nutrition that I deferred an internship for six months after graduation in order to work full time in her laboratory as a volunteer. This is an experience I have never forgotten and have always appreciated as a building block in forming the person I would become as time passed and as these events evolved. Good friendships were also made in the laboratory and carried on into life after medical school despite the many complications caused by a world standing at the abyss of the second World War.

There was an opportunity to develop friendships in Medical School. Each of us seemed to "bond" with a modest number of fellow students because of common interests or the joy of new experiences. Among my friends were Karl R. Paley, a friendship founded by alphabetical proximity of names and also by the warmth of good chemistry between us.

Other friends were Leroy Vandam who later became the Chairman of Anesthesiology at the Harvard affiliate, The Peter Bent Brigham Hospital. It is now the Brigham and Women's Hospital. The endowed anesthesiology chair there is named jointly for him and Benjamin Covino. Another anesthesiologist to be, also educated at Pennsylvania under the direction of Bob Dripps (as was Vandam) was Philip Sechser, later to be Chairman of Anesthesiology at Maimonides Medical Center in Brooklyn. Montague Ullman began his interest, psychiatry, in Medical School and became prominent in that field later. Then there was Jonas Salk, the conqueror of poliomyelitis about whom very much has already been said by others. He was a good friend in school and for years afterward.

INTERNSHIP AND RESIDENCY

Dr. Ralli urged me to remain at New York University and intern at Bellevue Hospital which I did with very great pleasure and happiness [despite the hard life all of us led].

To say that life at Bellevue Hospital was hard was a gross understatement despite all the interesting things that happened. Food was limited in quality and in volume for all of the Bellevue house officers of that period. We lived in a dormitory or multiple room type of set up in an old building which was known, accurately, as "Pneumonia Alley." I understood from my experiences what the word intern and resident meant. They were literal in those days. I do not believe I am exaggerating when I say that I don't recall having left the hospital even for a short time for a full six months. Our work load was enormous, our teaching was very effective and very good. It was a time of old fashioned courtesies and behavior patterns between doctors and of doctors with patients.

I remember for instance, going to the front door of the hospital dressed in a newly starched white uniform to greet the attending physician every day. I took his hat and coat and umbrella or a cane, to be sure that these were put away comfortably. I escorted him to the rounds which took place on the wards every morning in the early hours. Nobody thought that this was an imposition. In fact it was viewed as a privilege to be able to make these trips and, for a few minutes, to be in the presence alone with the "great man." Much was learned, many unusual things happened. [Syphilis was the AIDS of its time with all the same pejorative commentary that one can hear today.]

The experience at Bellevue included more than medicine. One night at about 2:00 a.m., I received a frantic call from the nurse in charge of the ward. I could not follow what had happened since she was almost hysterical. I went to the ward as quickly as I could and found an incredible scene of mayhem. A favorite cardiac patient of mine had evidently gone berserk. He seized the fire axe which hung in its designated place on the wall and then began a systematic attack on other patients. Blood was all over, on the floor, on beds and on the nurses' uniforms. I told the nurse to call the police and the psychiatrist on call. What to do next?

Somehow in the still of the night, disrupted by the violence of the axe attack, one could be either courageous or very stupid. It depends on how it turns out. The same act can be a "smashing" success or a dismal failure depending on the result.

I went up to Mr. X, with whom I had an excellent relationship and asked him for the axe. He relaxed, thought for a very long minute or two, and handed it to me. He went peacefully with the psychiatrist who had arrived to a secured ward in the Department of Psychiatry.

As fortune or luck would have it, the next phase in my life at Bellevue had the effect of career determination for me. My future teacher and one of the great pioneers in Anesthesiology,

E.A. Rovenstine, was the Head of the Anesthesiology service at Bellevue Hospital. He had arrived in New York City from Madison, Wisconsin some five years prior to the next incident that I wish to describe. There were rotations through the Anesthesiology service by surgical and medical house officers and since I had belonged to Medicine I was more or less eligible although it was not contemplated by the Faculty in the Department of Medicine that I should be placed on this rotation. Surgically oriented house officers usually were posted to anesthesiology.

However the person who was scheduled to go, came down with tuberculosis and required time for treatment in the famous Trudeau Sanitarium to facilitate his "cure." The Chief Resident in Medicine asked me in such a way that there was no possibility of my declining to accept being a substitute for him. I was assigned to join the anesthesiology service for one month's rotation in his place. I did this quite reluctantly because I was in the middle of some interesting work in Dr. Ralli's laboratory and felt that this was an unfair imposition not designed for my benefit and education. In a much more authoritarian age there was nothing to do but accept the assignment and reckon that one month would pass more or less quickly and that would be the end of it. However, much to my absolute surprise, the rotation though anesthesiology was tremendously exciting. I saw possibilities of important clinical care of people who were very sick. I had the great opportunity of working with surgeons and physicians from the three universities who at that time were in charge of three of the four divisions at Bellevue Hospital, i.e. New York University, Cornell and Columbia. The intensity of the operating room, the important role, as I viewed it, that one could play in being responsible for the life and well being of a patient were tremendously attractive. A flame seemed to have been lit up in me in a way that I did not expect.

Also, I had the desire to learn more about research strategy and technology. It seemed to me that anesthesiology lent itself particularly well to a research program that studied the impact of very powerful chemicals and drugs upon various systems in man. Having had the appropriate medical and research training for its time and after much soul searching and thinking about it I decided that I wanted to study anesthesiology and to do it in the best possible program that I could find. It was a revolutionary act for me. I went to see Dr. Rovenstine who had been very good to me even though he [at that time] thought I was to be there for only one month, to get his advice about what I should do. When one looks back and thinks about the brashness and the temerity of my approach, it is astonishing that I didn't have the sense to realize that what I was doing was something ridiculous. Perhaps the P&S Admissions Committee were quite right about my needing more time to mature! I had learned that the Department of Anesthesia at Wisconsin under the direction of Dr. Rovenstine's teacher and great friend, Dr. Ralph M. Waters, was the Mecca for anesthesiology education and I wanted to enlist his help in going there. To this day I do not realize how, why, and when the conversation changed but I found myself desirous of staying with Rovenstine and hoped to acquire all the things that could be gained with Waters in Wisconsin.

Needless to say my family and closest friends were all disappointed that I wasn't going to become either a Park Avenue internist or to continue my education to do research on medical problems concerning disease and its cure. Rovenstine had no room for me immediately and wanted me to defer my residency by spending a year working with the very distinguished physiologist at New York University and one of the world's experts on the function of the kidney, Dr. Homer W. Smith. Thus persuaded now by my second medical mentor to defer the next phase, I happened again by major serendipity to have had the privilege of learning from one of the truly greatest scientists in the world and of making friends with other people in his department, such as Dr. James A. Shannon who was to become the Director of the National Institutes of Health at a time crucial for this nation and very important for Anesthesiology and for me. This story will be told later.

Professor Homer W. Smith was the giant of renal physiology and a delightful and eloquent writer. He brought quantitative measurement from his strong background in physical chemistry to the determination of the various aspects of kidney functions including glomerular filtration, tubular function and the hemo-dynamics of the renal circulation. In addition to establishing a powerful reputation and a highly deserved one in this field, Smith also was interested in clinical application of his research. He was not medically qualified but he enjoyed working with a very able group of clinicians headed by Dr. William Goldring and Dr. Herbert Chasis at New York University and Bellevue Hospital's Department of Medicine to carry out studies [of this nature] on both healthy volunteers and patients with kidney, circulatory and cardiovascular diseases. It was a brilliant epoch in this aspect of life science.

Smith's laboratory attracted the kinds of people that so distinguished a leader would find interesting to develop. There was a mixture of people in basic science usually with a Ph.D. degree. The medically qualified individuals included the brilliant James Shannon, Sam Standard, Stanley Bradley the future Bard Professor of Medicine at Columbia and me among several others.

Smith assigned me to work with Stanley Bradley and Jim Shannon. All of this experience proved to be extremely valuable in many ways especially in guiding me further to the strategies of very good science and to the opportunities of making quantitative measurements in man as well as animals about events which take place during anesthesia. There was a very heady and exciting time for the person I was and the one into which I think I was evolving. There was excellent collaboration between Smith and Rovenstine which made life extremely good and interesting for me since I was a student of both. Later during my residency with Rovenstine, I remained a part time member of the Department of Physiology with Smith and helped in the teaching of laboratory science and physiological theory as well as continuing the research with Bradley which was to be taken up once again when we met later at Columbia's College of Physicians and Surgeons. Our collaborations, begun in Smith's department, continued at the Columbia Presbyterian-Medical Center after 1949 where we studied and succeeded in improving our understanding of kidney and hepatic function during various kinds of anesthesia and surgical operation. We were able to establish that there were certain automatic and autonomous functions in both systems. We could describe with reasonable accuracy the functions of both organs in response to the administration of different important anesthetic agents.

While maintaining this double program of an anesthesiology residency with a research career in physiology, there was very little time for other activities including taking advantage of the social and intellectual aspects of the great city of New York. However, it was all worth while and if I had the opportunity of repeating it I would want it very little different from my actual experience.

When I became one of Rovenstine's residents a similar experience of outstanding individuals was evident. John Adriani was still in New York at Bellevue. Stuart Cullen had recently left to assume the directorship of the division at the University of Iowa. Mary Lou Byrd was a chief resident at a time when women were very rarely so placed and was getting ready to make her mark in Grand Rapids, Michigan. Ralph Sappenfield was getting ready to go to Florida. Sydney Lyons was finishing as a senior resident and brought the Rovenstine brand of anesthesiology to the Mount Sinai Hospital in New York. Charles Burstein, who did so much to advance cardiac surgery and anesthesia during World War II, had gone to the Hospital for Special Surgery. Solomon Hershey had joined a year after I did and prepared himself for his future brilliant career of heading the Beth Israel Department of Anesthesiology. Louis Orkin was part of the group, an experience which prepared him for his distinguished career at Albert Einstein in New York.

The clinical experience with Rovenstine was wonderful in its excellence. At the time of my residency, he was a great teacher and a marvelous clinician who was highly respected by all of the surgeons in the three university divisions at Bellevue. He made a major impact on anesthesiological practice in New York City by bringing the Waters message of excellent science supporting and modifying clinical practice for the benefit of patients. The Monday night clinical meetings and clinical case presentations that were part of Rovenstine's teaching exercises were open to all anesthesiologists and other interested people in the city of New York. They were most informative and were clearly exciting. They were given at 8:00 p.m. in a big auditorium at Bellevue and Rovenstine presided over them in charismatic fashion. These were the most important teaching experiences in anesthesiology in New York City and possibly in the country at large. It was not competitively possibly for other anesthesiologists to bring that type of leadership and knowledge of science and clinical practice to bear in so splendid a fashion. Rovenstine may have been light years ahead of his time in this regard.

His presence had made such an impression on the New York scene in anesthesiology and its related clinical fields that he attracted widespread attention in the press. Magazine articles were written about him. He was also an important and frequent guest speaker at important medical meetings throughout this country and the rest of the world. This magic of his personality and his contributions were captured in a three part profile in the New Yorker magazine during the time that I was with him. The three part profile is a *must* reading for people who want to understand more of the nature of this man and his major accomplishments in so many different aspects of the world that he dominated. His mid-western origins were fully described. The writer, Mark Murphy, practically lived with Rovey for about six weeks in order to get not only the essential information about him but to watch him in action and to understand some of the subtleties of a very special and also a very complicated human being. Murphy did this job very well and all of the important characteristics of the man are mentioned, often analyzed and always put in reasonable perspective to his character and his accomplishments.

However, the articles about him in the New Yorker caused a considerable amount of upheaval in his life and in mine. He was suspended from the New York County Medical Society for unethical behavior and self aggrandizement. The notion in the early 1940's when the profiles appeared was that no physician should be featured in an article in the media including the public press and radio because it was considered to be advertising which was believed to lead to monetary benefit to the person who permitted it.

After Rovey's suspension from the New York County Society for one year he was considered ineligible for participation in any of organized medicine's venues including, of course, the meetings of the American Medical Association. Rovey and I had written a paper together. He was the senior author and was scheduled to present it at the annual meeting of the AMA in Chicago. We were very upset that he was ruled ineligible by the officers of the Section on Anesthesiology to present our paper. They offered a compromise in that I would be permitted to present the paper despite having been censured by the New York County Medical Society for being mentioned in the profile of Rovey in a minor role. Rovey and I attempted to get in touch with Dr. Waters who was his close friend and his mentor to come to Chicago to help mediate the dispute. Unfortunately for us, Dr. Waters was on vacation in Door County and felt that it wasn't necessary for him to come. We understood his feelings yet differed with him because it was our firm conviction that his over riding presence and his support of Rovey would carry the day comfortably. In any event this did not occur and when the paper was announced at the meeting and that I would present it, I came up to the podium and, with Rovey's full approval, tried to tell the story of how Rovey was being barred unreasonably, in our view, from the opportunity to present the paper as originally scheduled. I was ruled out of order by the Chair and this ruling prevailed. The paper therefore was never presented and as I left the meeting, very unhappy at the outcome, I was stopped by another young person who was destined to become one of my closest friends, Albert Faulconer, a member of the Mayo Clinic staff. He stopped me, having heard of the dispute on the podium, and said he wanted to know me better because I was either one of the most courageous people he ever met or I was one damned fool to end my career so precipitously over an issue that in due course would not loom to be of importance. Therefore, from my point of view, one of the very good things that happened as a by product of the behavior that I have just described was the close and warm friendship of a man with a fabulous mind and equally wonderful personality. In the long list of things of importance I would say that if the encounter with the AMA was necessary to establish a friendship with Albert Faulconer, it was worth all of the storm and unpleasantness.

Rovey was an expert teacher in the classical sense of that term. He was incredibly fetching and persuasive as a speaker. However, he had an unusual attitude about speaking in a lecture format. He thought that audiences would think that he was either ill prepared or not prepared if he used his skills in an obvious way as a lecturer. If the subject was well known to him, as was usually the case, he could speak extemporaneously without a single note or text and the lecture would come out highly polished, elegant and clear to all those who listened. This was an incredibly fabulous gift that he had. Because of his attitude about audiences it was never fully appreciated. For instance what he often did was have me put together a folder with blank pages in it which he would turn from time to time while lecturing and pretended to look at the text which didn't exist so that the audience would be persuaded that he really had worked to prepare the material. Besides he was quite presbyopic and could not read without eyeglasses. I was much amused by this quirk of his but it was no laughing matter to him. It was not a subject about which it was permissible to joke. One of the by-products for me was the realization that if the lecture could be given as magnificently as he did, the audience would be captured even if he used no notes and perhaps would be even more impressed. There are many people who have such abilities and they extend into other fields as well. Listening to a concert, when a conductor does not use a score has always impressed me as being an unusual feat. The same reaction goes when a splendid lecture is given without notes or text. There is of course the alternative of using slides allegedly for the illumination of concepts to the audience but really as a common source of reminders for the lecturer as well as guidance for the audience. I have tried sometimes quite successfully to give lectures in this form and have even dared a few times to do it without slides or without any visible material other than my understanding of what it is that I wanted to say. All this I learned from a splendid lecturer like Rovey.

He was, long before it was commonplace, very much interested in regional anesthesia and its potential use for the alleviation of pain of various types. He came to Bellevue at the time when the memory of the very distinguished French surgeon who was expert in regional anesthesia, Gaston Labat, had favorably impressed New York medicine. At this point a brief diversion to Dr. Labat might be of interest. The point arises when one wonders why Gaston Labat would have been at Bellevue Hospital shortly before Rovenstine's appearance there and what influence he might have had upon Rovey?

The story, perhaps somewhat apocryphal, was that one of the Mayo brothers had met Labat in Paris and was so impressed by his great skills at regional anesthesia that he invited him to the Mayo clinic to do this type of anesthesia for surgery. Labat, a surgeon, developed regional anesthesia to a very high degree of excellence and wrote a magnificent textbook on the subject. The story proceeds further. When Dr. Labat arrived at the Mayo clinic he was accompanied by a different lady than the Madame Labat that Dr. Mayo had met in Paris. Apparently this upset Dr. Mayo because he did not want to have an "immoral" relationship at the Mayo clinic. Labat was asked to leave. Rather than return to France directly he came to Bellevue in New York invited by people who knew of his work, including another surgeon in New York, Dr. H. Wertheim who was also very good at regional anesthesia. Wertheim maintained a very busy surgical practice. Dr. Wertheim became a close friend of Rovenstine's and probably taught him some of the regional anesthesia that he may have acquired from Labat. Undoubtedly the legacy of Labat's contribution to regional anesthesia at Bellevue as well as Dr. Wertheim's skill and interest were important factors in stimulating Dr. Rovenstine's activity in this subject. Mme. Labat gave Rovenstine the plates of a projected second edition of Labat's classical book on Regional Anesthesia which was not completed because of Labat's untimely death. Unfortunately, Rovenstine was not a writer of books. He never wrote the Labat second edition. The plates disappeared and to my knowledge were never found.

There were very many limitations for nerve blocks. The armamentarium of drugs for successful and controllable nerve blocks was very limited. Needles were not as useful in the early 1940s as they are now. There were no plastic catheters. However, Rovey's brilliance and ability to see far in to the future overcame a good many of these objections [at least to a reasonable degree]. For example, he established the first pain clinic that actually functioned for patient care in this country. He used nerve block for anesthesia for surgical procedures with considerable skill. He also, as always, wanted to share the knowledge that he had acquired by teaching this subject of regional anesthesia both for surgical operations as well as the management of pain. He developed a course, short in duration, that combined anatomical dissection of cadavers, seminars, lectures and practical demonstrations with patients of this very new and exciting field. People came from many parts of the country to learn because of his very powerful reputation as an educator as well as a clinician and scientist. The distinguished Chairman of Anesthesiology at the University of Pennsylvania, Dr. Robert D. Dripps and some of his associates Doctors Austin Lamont, James Eckenhoff and Leroy Vandam were also students in that course.

This activity in the management of pain with regional anesthesia also had an impact on the non-medical world. Reporters and photographers from Life Magazine wanted to put together a pictorial story of the therapy of pain with nerve block. There was a very large spread in an issue of Life Magazine and it created quite a lot of attention for the subject as well as for Rovenstine and for me. I was featured in the main photograph. A small memento was given to me by Rovey shortly thereafter when I was called up as a reserve officer to enter the Army of the United States. This was a gold spinal needle that had belonged to and was used by Dr. Gaston Labat for spinal anesthesia and had found its way in to Rovenstine's possession as a gift from Labat or his widow. It is one of the important pieces of equipment that I have cherished all the years since then because it has so noble an anesthesiological history and provenance.

The life with Rovenstine and Smith was a heady and exciting one. However, it could not be denied that things were in a very serious state in our world. War had broken out in Europe. To many of us it seemed inevitable that we would be drawn into the conflict or elect to enter it. Plans were being made as to what we should do in preparation. Rovenstine who had served in World War I wanted very much to participate in the Armed Forces in World War II. He would have been an outstanding choice to direct anesthesia activities in any of the theaters of operation or to do what needed most to be done to develop manpower in anesthesiology. Whatever the reason, Rovey's wishes were never fulfilled and he was not part of the military effort but he was a major figure in teaching young physicians who had had the curtailed three year medical education of the war period and a nine month internship, by providing them with opportunities to learn something about anesthesiology. These three year and nine month "wonders" were an important part of our war effort because well educated well trained people in anesthesiology for the Armed Forces did not exist in adequate numbers.

It was generally thought that there were no more than fifty completely trained and educated anesthesiologists by the standards of 1941 and 1942. These skills had to be vastly extended in a way that provided for safe anesthetic management of our soldiers, sailors and airmen who became casualties of the war.

The fact that it turned out so well was a tribute to many including those who stayed behind like Rovenstine and Lundy to do the teaching as well as to senior medical military officers who provided the very sympathetic support in all the branches of the medical military services. The military leadership in anesthesiology provided by Drs. Beecher, McCuskey and Tovell in our various overseas theaters of operation was outstanding.

MARRIAGE AND FAMILY

The description of my activities in medical school and residency have sounded very much as though there was no family or social life whatever. However there was enough time to form a happy relationship which resulted in my marriage to Julia Fisher.

We had met inevitably because of her being in the Class of 1937 at Barnard College just across the street from Columbia College at Morningside Heights. She was two years behind me in academic work. We met at a party at which some of the undergraduate students at Columbia and at Barnard were present and we took to each other rather quickly. It was 1939, war was destined to break out in Europe in the early fall. It gave a sense of urgency to many young people and we were no exceptions. Since I was already a reserve officer, it was unlikely that I would not be among the early ones called should we enter the conflict.

I knew Julia's brother, Saul Fisher, who was two years ahead of me in the School of Medicine at New York University, because he also worked in Homer Smith's laboratory. His work on the tubular reabsorption phenomena of the human kidney was significant and interesting. Although we knew each other, it was not a close friendship in that our paths were somewhat differently shaded by political affairs since he was much more to the left than I was in those days. It wan no surprise to discover that so was Julia, but then so were many young people at that time, interested in seeing a better world than the mixed up chaotic and destructive one which we seemed to be living in. The Roosevelt "revolution" had made such beliefs acceptable and to some extent even quite popular among thinking young people. In fact, I was viewed as somewhat of a peculiar one since I had not gone along with the total belief that the Soviet Union reflected a good future whereas much of the rest of Europe was in the grips of monstrous fascists. It seemed desirable to most of them and somehow not to me that we should go in that direction. Even though I recognized all the many inequalities and inequities that were driving them that way I could not take the last steps because I still believed that it was possible, and the Roosevelt Administration was showing that it was, to have the American way evolve and develop to accommodate to the needs of the future.

As this piece is being written in 1996 it seems that my prognostication was only partially correct. The caring for others attitude of the New Deal is now being challenged and the welfare state being junked, for what form of government remains to be seen. Despite our political differences, Julia and I got along extremely well. After a brief but intensive courtship we were married in a way that suited both our families. There was a big wedding. It was white tie and tails, and she looked wonderful in her bridal gown. We were married on December 21, 1939 as I was finishing my training in Internal Medicine before beginning my research fellowship in physiology. I had worked several consecutive nights for my friends and colleagues in the house staff rotation so that I could have a few days off for a honeymoon. Youth is never to be denied, I guess, because I seemed to have been able to get married and have a pleasant honeymoon on very little sleep for those few days after December 21. Our wedding day ended in the longest night in the year for whatever that might mean!

Julia had, just prior to our marriage, obtained a very interesting position on the secretarial staff to President Roosevelt and was assigned, for some of that time to the Women's Division of the Democratic National Committee where she got to know very many important people including Mrs. Roosevelt and the President. Even though this was long before the days of the feminist revolution, I felt that her job was much more important than mine. I felt it was my responsibility to try to secure a position in Washington where she was living and stationed rather than to attempt to have her give up her job and come to New York. Another possibility was for us stay where we were and commute when it was feasible to do so. That, at first, did not occur to us but it eventuated for the next year or so while I was a research fellow with Homer Smith. I never got a position in Washington that was acceptable to me and approved by her nor did she wish to move to New York for something less exciting and wonderful than working for the President and Mrs. Roosevelt. Our solution consisted of my commuting from New York to Washington and I did it as often as things allowed. Actually I got to Washington perhaps twice a month or even less frequently during that year but our marriage thrived because of the interesting work we were both doing and the fact that we knew that at some point in time things would change. She was committed, other things being equal (which they weren't) to stay through the President's second term and into the third term since, a year after we were married, he would be elected to a third term in that high office for the first time in American history.

My visits to Washington were fascinating. Very often I would either be met or have a message at the train station in Washington for me to proceed to one or another sights in Washington. The message usually read that Miss Fisher was not available until X hours later. I therefore saw a great many of the important sights in Washington during the period when the war had begun in Europe and had not yet involved us in the United States.

Julia lived with four friends in a very nice apartment on Connecticut avenue in Washington which had one regular bedroom and several other makeshift devices for the ladies to take turns in where they slept. When I came down, she and I were given the one bedroom they had and I was looked after almost like a young princeling by these wonderful roommates of hers. Those friendships that she made lasted a very long time for both of us and it was a very exciting time indeed for her and vicariously for me. Among the interesting things that happened to me apart from the sight seeing and the excitement of Washington was that an occasional Sunday night supper prepared by Mrs. Roosevelt at the White House included me. I had the happy experience of being totally ignored except as "Ms. Fisher's husband" but I was able uninterruptedly and without being disturbed to watch the magnificent and interesting activities of carrying the President down on his chair when he made no pretense of being able to stand or walk and to listen to the brilliant and lively discussion that went on around me. It was a moving and exhilarating experience for both of us and certainly enlarged my horizons more than I ever expected would be possible. I also learned a lesson about the role of women. Equality with men was necessary for them. I learned that they deserved any position that merit could support. After the exciting year in Washington and just before I was called up to active duty in the Army, Julia moved back to New York. She was appointed the first full time Executive Director of the New York State League of Women Voters where she was able to continue to exert serious influence on the political process.

Some of the personal matters in our marriage need to be mentioned. Our having a family was based mostly on emergency military leaves because my mother at the time was suffering from what was thought to be a fatal illness. She had aplastic anemia of unknown origin and twice I was called back to New York for an emergency visit because it was thought that she was perilously near death. These emergency leaves resulted in two pregnancies, our daughter Barbara and our son Richard.

In addition, Julia and I had to settle our affairs early on and deal with the problems of many new relationships, including, attempting to and succeeding in making new friends in Miami. So active were we in this regard that possibly some of the subtle effects of Julia's oncoming illness were not apparent to her or to me. Whatever the reason she began to be noticeably ill in 1973 and when first diagnosed after a rapid work up it was found that she had a cancer of the body of the pancreas with metastases already present in the liver and the lungs when the diagnosis was first made. It was a shattering blow in every respect for me. Our children were very solicitous for both of us. Dick was in Law School at Yale and paid as much attention to us as he had time. He was very good and very strong about this. Barbara had Andy, who was born in 1971 and was very busy with the new baby and her husband, Bill who was now a medical student in Miami after having earned a Ph.D. in Physics in Columbia. It was very important for Julia to be able to be with Andy and enjoy him while he was still an infant. As the illness progressed she became weaker and weaker and the time of being able to cope was fast disappearing. As her health continued to fail, the children did all they could to be close to me and to her and finally she could no longer hold out. Tender loving care was given to her by our physician, Dr. Chester Cassel. Another person who provided what she could during Julia's final days was Elaine Blumenthal. I did the best I could. She died on the 6th of March, 1974 and there was terrible devastation for me, for the children and, although he was too small to know it, for Andy. It was two days before Barbara's thirtieth birthday.

I spent much of the remainder of 1974 in mourning and tried to work as best I could at the tough job at the School of Medicine at the University of Miami that still needed to be done. The work was in some way a life saver in that I was able to concentrate on my job in the Dean's office. I could overcome, while working, elements of the terrible tragedy that had happened to me. During that time I spent some weekends in London and some in New York just to go to the theater where I could lose myself in forgetfulness.

Perhaps ordained by Fate working its mysterious way in magical fashion, I was invited to Elaine and Sidney Blumenthal's apartment in Key Biscayne for what I thought would be a pleasant Sunday night supper for the three of us. I walked over to the Blumenthal's from my home on that Sunday night which happened to be June 2nd of 1974 needing a shave, in shorts and sandals, and not even close to being attractive looking at all.

Much to my surprise and early negative reaction there were several other people there of whom Patricia Goldstein was one. I did not know at the time but learned very quickly thereafter that the Blumenthals and their close friends, the Hills, who were good friends of Pat's had apparently made an arrangement between them to see that the two of us were to meet and hopefully would be attracted to each other to develop a meaningful relationship possibly even one of marriage. They could not have been more correct in their judgment and to this day, and probably forever, I will be grateful to all four of them for doing what they did to bring us together.

Two things had happened. The first of these was Pat's separation and subsequent divorce from Charles Goldstein and the second was my being widowed in March of 1974. The timing was fortuitous. Pat, I think, was ready for a new relationship perhaps reluctantly so but unconsciously ready. It turned out for me that I was more than ready and was absolutely delighted to finally feel that I once again wished to be alive in this world and to live to the fullest. She was almost magical in providing a desire for me to lift the depression under which I had suffered for quite a few months and to once again want to rejoin the world and its people. We hit it off very well that night. A great transformation had taken place in me. I began to get more optimistic. I wanted to do things and I certainly wanted to be with her. I pursued this prospective new relationship with Pat with vigor and with happiness. I had the support of my children in wanting to make a new life for myself. Perhaps they were getting a bit tired of having to worry about me and my depressed demeanor but whatever it was they were positive in suggesting that this would be a happy and very good relationship for me. We saw a good deal of each other in the subsequent months and when her divorce became final and all arrangements completed we decided to marry and that was done with great happiness for both of us on the last day of November of 1975.

That marriage has been an extraordinary one and I cannot figure out exactly how I got to be so lucky as to have two ladies who were willing to marry me in two different times in my life who couldn't be more different and yet who were absolutely wonderful in their respective and differing ways. I owe Pat my life and much of my happiness. She has made an enormous difference in keeping me happy, healthy and I am almost tempted to say wise!

WORLD WAR II

When the war began in Europe in 1939 it seemed clear to me and to many of my friends that it was inevitable that the United States would be drawn into this conflict. It was, in a way, a reaffirmation of a world fast approaching chaos. Europe was in flames and had to impact America sooner or later. Since many of us are of European descent there always is an immediacy about conflict and trouble in Europe. Our position as a major world power was also an important factor. Japan's expansionist aggressions started long before the war in Europe because of her behavior motivated by "Bushido" or military power to achieve economic and political dominance in Asia. Although just as difficult and as ominous as anything in Europe it was not Europe and it did not seem to concern most Americans in the same way as the confrontation in Europe did.

I felt strongly about the values of our American society which had made possible so many opportunities for me and also for my family. I believed that it was my duty to enlist and I did so as a reserve officer in the Army. Also there was clear cut evidence to most of us that this would be a total societal effort which would be reflected in the mobilization of industry, manufacturing, economic strength and creative intelligence. It appeared as though there would be a mobilization of a size and a persuasiveness that this country had never before realized. In short it was a total effort in a cause that was largely accepted by most Americans even though there were conspicuous dissenters.

There were many decisions possible for a person of my age, a physician with educational and practical experience in internal medicine, anesthesiology and scientifically in physiology. I felt that I might have a place in the Armed Forces because of these professional skills and my excellent state of health except for a long-lasting and lingering experience with migraine which caused no important disability but did occasionally result in ophthalmoplegic episodes I therefore decided to apply for a commission in the reserves of the Army of the United States when I was twenty four years old. I was accepted and experienced the bustle of all the "paperwork" which was necessary to complete the reserve enlistment. I was erroneously assigned to the Artillery but was not aware of this situation.

After the Japanese attack on Pearl Harbor, December 7, 1941, (as President Roosevelt characterized it "a day that will live in infamy") I knew that my being called to active duty would be relatively soon after our rapid entry into the war in the Pacific against Japan and in Europe against Germany. I was called to active duty soon enough but it took a few months in the confusion of that time for efficient processing of the American mobilization to take place. I received orders to report two different places at nearly the same time. I asked for transfer from the Artillery to the medical corps which was immediately granted although it took some time to effect. My dual assignment was also corrected. All of this eventually was straightened out and I finally reported in June, 1942 to a new temporary Army General Hospital in Palm Springs, California. The institution was named after a former medical military officer. It was known at that time as Torney General Hospital. The hospital had to be newly constructed except for the space occupied by the former El Mirador Hotel which was taken over by the Army for the development of this general hospital. It was to be used in support of the Desert Training Center for the Army's Armored Force based in Indio, California, a small town near Palm Springs. The medical staff, who were collected at Torney General Hospital, had no patients in the first few months. It was dreadfully hot in the summer time. In order to keep our sanity as the hospital was being built and as the Tank Units were appearing in the desert for training, we kept ourselves busy by helping the construction people build the hospital and we got to know each other better in that capacity. It was an exceedingly uncomfortable experience actually participating in the construction of a hospital in one of the hottest climates that I had experienced up to that time.

The hospital was constructed quickly and eventually admitted patients who were in the Armored Divisions in training in the desert for future combat in Europe, Africa and presumably the Pacific theater as well.

I served as Chief of Anesthesiology and controlled the operating room facilities as well. Because of my internal medical education, when we were not operating I also served as a Staff Officer of the Officer's ward. I was commissioned prior to my call to active duty as a First Lieutenant in the Army Medical Corps. I was quickly promoted to Captain, which seemed to be consistent with the responsibilities I had acquired. Many friendships among the medical officers and their enlisted men were formed that lasted a good many years and persisted into the post war period. It was an interesting experience. This was my first activity in which I was in charge of something and working with surgeons of considerable ability who had never seen the kind of modern anesthesia that the Wisconsin School and its leaders Doctors Waters and Rovenstine had been preaching in the civilian world. All of this made for a very happy professional experience. I certainly enjoyed also the opportunity to practice internal medicine with commissioned officers many of whom had illnesses acquired in the Pacific theater and were sent to us for treatment or convalescence. It was at this institution that I had the very great pleasure of starting Jim West and Sam Denson on a career in anesthesiology which was eventually to become their lifelong profession. These fifty four years later I still see Jim West from time to time and am always saddened by the remembrance of the death of Sam Denson.

Later, I had a brief assignment in northern California at Dibble General Hospital in Menlo Park, not far from Stanford University in Palo Alto and of course near San Francisco. The assignment was a very pleasant and very busy one working with the earliest of returning war casualties from the Pacific theater. We performed a great deal of reconstructive surgery for war wounds. We had a very large hand and orthopedic service. We were also a major center for plastic repair of all sorts of war wounds including eye injuries.

I had the opportunity of doing a substantial number of regional anesthetic procedures for the hand service and also for the orthopedic and plastic services. Essentially, except for the injuries and the war wounds, the patients were young healthy men. It was a marvelously gratifying experience for us who took care of them. It could never have occurred in any civilian hospital since it was the massive numbers of patients and the need to move them along as quickly as possible that made our experience possible. We were rated for fifteen hundred beds and always were full. We usually had another fifteen hundred patients who were out of the hospital and returning periodically for staged operations of one sort or another. My clinical experience was very greatly broadened in these two institutions and I very much cherish and value it in retrospect as well as having enjoyed it at the time.

In due course, in the early part of 1944, I was transferred overseas to the European theater of operations in the early part of 1944. It was still winter and the change from northern California to the United Kingdom, north of London was not exactly a happy experience in terms of the weather. However the military medical story was very different. I was temporarily assigned to the Eighth Air Force Base at Lakenheath just north of London. One must remember that there was no separate American Air Force during World War II and that it was part of the Army. During this period I got to know many of the personnel who were based there. Those I knew best were a heavy bombardment group (the aircraft was the B-17, otherwise known as the Flying Fortress) I felt greatly concerned, as an observer without flight surgical training, at the exposure to injury and death of these young and very brave flyers each time they flew sorties against "Fortress Europe." I was deeply worried about their welfare and tried to learn more about what could be done to improve their chances of staying alive as well as dealing with the consequences of stress and anxiety [that is] occasioned in many people — probably most — because of the nature of the combat flying experience. I knew full well that highly competent experts were working on this tough problem and recognized that my ability consisted only in compassion and not in skill.

The personnel in most instances were rather young men, extremely fit and very brave in my opinion. However they did what seemed to me to be stupid things. When they returned from a sortie over Europe it was common for many of them to drink too much, to sleep too little and to spend excessive amounts of time in sexual and other social carousing which certainly diminished their ability to concentrate and be safe when they flew their next missions, usually without much opportunity to rest. When I discussed this with one of the wing commanders, purely as a friend, which I was until my regular assignment came through, he invited me to fly with him on a routine mission over the English Channel into Western Europe to get some idea of what it was like. Therefore, without appropriate orders or any useful knowledge, I accepted the invitation and once we were aloft he told me that because of security he could not previously inform me that the mission had changed. We were going to attack a major German ball bearing factory that was likely to be very heavily defended. The consequences of this bombing mission would be a high casualty rate for our aircraft and therefore its personnel. He apologized to me for what he described as a "major inconvenience to me."

My friend's predictions were unfortunately only too accurate. We very quickly found ourselves in a hailstorm of anti-aircraft fire and German fighter planes. I had no training in evacuation from damaged aircraft but I was wearing a parachute as was required. We were severely hit and all of the people in our airplane were evacuated via parachute. I remember that I was pushed out on the orders of the Captain and apparently the parachute must have opened automatically or some other way because I did not know how to use one. I landed successfully but was injured in both shoulders, the abdomen and the chest.

Young teenagers who worked in the Resistance were there to pick up those of us who survived the landings. They took us through the south of France, across its border with Spain which was a neutral country and into neutral Portugal. We were transported carefully and quietly at night and handed over from one resistance group to another until most of our survivors made it into Portugal after what seemed like an eternity of time but probably was something of the order of ten days to two weeks. I have considerable amnesia for this period and only know that I was operated upon somewhere in France and was in a shoulder and arm splint until we arrived in Portugal. We were then transported safely to England when our physical condition permitted. It was a horrifying experience which I found impossible to even talk about for some thirty five years after it occurred. Some minor revision of the first shoulder operation had to be done and then I was judged fit for the resumption of my medical duties in due course. The other injuries healed without operation, but a big diaphragmatic hernia remained. Survivors of this experience were all decorated with either the bronze or the silver star and there were few indeed. I was promoted to the rank of Major. Instead, therefore, of facing what I had thought would be a court martial for being absent without leave, I found myself a decorated officer who was promoted for alleged gallantry in action!

After a suitable period of convalescence I was assigned to a position of Battalion Surgeon in General Patton's Third Army. All of this took place several weeks after the D-Day invasion of Normandy. The Third Army had broken out of St. Lo and was on its way eastward towards Paris. The resistance by the Germans in the early part of the rapid movement of this great army across north western France was heavy. The resistance was only broken further along as it became obvious that the Germans had comparably little air strength to harass the American force and insufficient infantry and armored force to be a major military factor.

In all these activities, mobility on the part of the American Tankers was essential, as had been very well proven by the Germans in the original Blitzkrieg which conquered the low countries and France.

However our wounded and killed were far from inconsequential in number. This was one of the first problems that had to be understood by young physicians who had recently been civilian officers and were now medical officers of the army. We were told repeatedly by the headquarters command, by personal communication to all service personnel (of which the medical department was a major one in warfare), that our responsibility in the military effort was to keep as many officers and soldiers fighting as was humanly possible. Very often this meant a reversal of the traditional American sense of ethics and of right and wrong. We were required in many instances to take care of the most lightly wounded and less seriously injured men first in order to return them to combat since that was necessary for the strength of the military advance across France. There were plenty of doctors who had difficulties with this reversal of ordinary civilian efforts and I certainly was one of them. However, I understood full well that success in warfare depended on the destruction of enemy forces and that could only be done by preserving as many of the fit and those who became fit by our efforts as it was possible to do. Probably soldiers were lost by this policy but one will never know how many. We did the best we could considering our skills and considering our sense of right and wrong but we conformed to the requirements of a very horrible and unpleasant period.

At one stage of the campaign because of my complete training in anesthesia I was moved from these duties of first contact with wounded and injured troops to a hospital setting where we had greater opportunity to treat surgical wounds in the way that we were accustomed to do. If they survived their initial wounding and injury we were not only permitted but encouraged to take as good care of them as we knew how.

I was very often the only person who had known anything about anesthesiology in the hospital. Occasionally there was a young Doctor who had had the nine months of internship which I have described earlier in the story. It became necessary to try to develop anesthetic methods that were as safe as possible and yet permitted important surgery and often quite difficult surgery to be performed under the most adverse of circumstances. The major factor operating in our favor was that our patients were strong, physically fit right up the moment of their injury or wounding. We had their constitutional capabilities and strengths going for them as well as for our efforts. I had also to try to multiply myself in many ways and decided to educate and train very intelligent enlisted corpsmen in one or more procedures so that I could go from patient to patient and do what had to be done. In these settings my knowledge often had to be spread over somewhere between five and twelve operating rooms and it was not an easy task. My decisions were based upon those realities. Very often I did as much regional anesthesia as I could consistent with the patients' conditions, emotional as well as physical. I taught these wondrous enlisted men how to take the blood pressure and measure other vital signs that could be used as indices for supplementary treatment, transfusion, or other medications. I also used a good deal of spinal anesthesia but made every effort to keep the height of the block below T-10 if that was consistent with the surgical requirements and the patient's condition. It is unnecessary to state the obvious. I became very good at regional procedures and was limited only by the characteristics of the local anesthetic drugs that had to be employed and were available to us. We had some difficulty in this regard because we had very few drugs and none of them with the characteristics providing long lasting block that could be manipulated with versatility.

For general anesthesia we had thiopental, nitrous oxide and ether. Often for these patients I chose an endotracheal airway and taught the enlisted men how to make observations assuming that I would be instantly available. I was always available for any problem that might have ensued. Actually my physical presence and my input into the management of all of these patients occurred almost every few minutes because I was going from room to room constantly to be sure that all the things that could be done were being done. Toward the end of this experience we received small amounts of relatively impure curare manufactured by the Squibb Company and known by their trade name, Intocostrin. It was used to great advantage.

What we did was to employ relatively modest doses of the muscle relaxant and supplement it with narcotics, using only nitrous oxide and oxygen towards the end of the surgical procedure. Our goal was to have patients who could be awake enough to move off the operating table themselves on to a chair or to a stretcher. It was a huge advance in safety for patients who had major surgical procedures. It turned out, of course, to be a crude precursor of the soon to be widely used non-potent anesthetic by inhalation reinforced by narcotics and supplemented by muscle relaxants. This method was developed to a high degree of excellence by Professor Gray and his colleagues in civilian life. They certainly deserve all the credit for organizing it reliably and reproducibly. My use of it was a simply an attempt to overcome a clinical problem. If the patient could be responsible for his own airway and respiratory functions it greatly increased safety and also sharply reduced the requirement for close and supervisory nursing care. We didn't have these capabilities at hand so this method proved to be extremely valuable.

All of these anesthetic experiences under combat conditions produced an extraordinary spurt of knowledge and creativity on the part of many who had to cope and deal with these problems. We certainly knew that we were in for a massive amount of change in our attitude and activities from those we had been accustomed to in civilian life. It is necessary also to mention that controlled respiration, while known in civilian life, was not used widely at first in warfare. There were very few useful respirators and at this stage none was available. I am not sure we would have been able to learn fast enough to use them with the skill of today. We also had very few precise monitoring devices beyond the ability to take the blood pressure, to count the pulse and to count the respiration. We learned fast enough how to estimate the adequacy or inadequacy of minute ventilation by clinical judgment.

After the end of the war in Europe on VE-Day in May of 1945 many of us were transferred back to the United States or directly to the Pacific theater to prepare for the final episodes of the war against Japan. Obviously nobody knew of the atomic weapons. The invasion of Japan was viewed as a military activity that would take many lives and injure many more.

I was transferred to the Walter Reed Hospital in Washington. This institution was a magnificent one and was the central flagship hospital of the regular army for a good many years. I felt particularly fortunate to be allowed to work as the Chief of Anesthesiology and Operating Rooms. I also was asked to help in some staff work at the Pentagon as were other officers who had the length of experience of young and reasonably healthy (except probably psychologically) medical officers like me. At Walter Reed Hospital the clinical experience was something of a hybrid between military and civilian types of anesthesia and surgery. There were many returning veterans whose wounds or injuries qualified them for release from the Armed Forces. There were others who were important in the military command and were stationed in Washington and needed care of one sort or another obtained at Walter Reed. Some who lived in or near the District of Columbia were also sent to that institution because of their particular abilities and requirements.

Anesthesia at this very large hospital was different. There were several junior people who had several months, usually three, of anesthesia training who could work with me and there were also nurse anesthetists usually in the regular Army. The practice was a very busy one for all of these reasons and a very illuminating and interesting one.

When VJ-Day came, unexpectedly to most of us, there was a great urge for as many of us as could arrange it, to be released from active duty and return to civilian life. I certainly had no desire to stay in the regular Army or in the Reserves and wanted to return to civilian status as soon as it was possible. With all my accumulated leave I was released from the Army in the winter of 1945 and officially discharged from the Army on April 1, 1946. This was no April Fool's Day! On that happy day I began seriously to try to sort out where I should be.

THE EARLY POST WAR PERIOD

At the end of World War II and after four years of military service, a whole new set of problems in living arose for me and I think for many of my contemporaries. We could not imagine a world without war and its dangers even though everybody hoped both consciously and unconsciously for the end of hostilities. We were unsettled as to what to do with the new challenge of once more becoming civilians and not subject to military oversight and rule over the location and nature of all our activities.

Like many of my good friends, I was worn out with the war. I yearned, at first, for a lovely and bucolic way of life after the war, to engage in a private practice in a small and lovely community, preferably in California and give up all of the notions of research, the intellectual excitement of the academic medical center and the career or careers in which I was engaged before the war. I was powerfully attracted to a life of comfort and devoid of conflict. I received an excellent offer to join good friends who were companions of mine in the Army to practice in Redlands, California, a lovely town approximately midway between Los Angeles and the desert town of Palm Springs. Meredith Beaver had been Chief of Surgery at my first military assignment in Palm Springs and we became close friends. We even wrote an article together on anesthesia for total gastrectomy. The reality of Redlands was different from my fantasies about it. When I revisited that serene town as a civilian at Dr. Beaver's invitation after he had returned to direct the Beaver Clinic in Redlands, I knew intuitively it was not for me. I began to be perplexed about what to do, since the yearning for a peaceful, beautiful climate even while working reasonably hard was not as appealing as it had been while I was still in the military service.

I was still attracted to the idea of a salubrious climate and and attempted to get a position at the University of California in San Francisco but was told by the Chairman of Anesthesiology that there were no vacancies and it was unlikely that there would be any in the future. The outstanding future growth and development of that splendid medical institution were not appreciated by all of those who were in control of activities at UCSF right after the end of the war. With the California possibilities not available or not desirable, I decided that I would return, if he would have me, to Rovenstine's department in New York and, in doing so, return to familiar territory, a very agreeable intellectual environment and the security of minimizing unknown factors. I therefore rejoined him and was welcomed with open arms, much to my delight, even though it was no surprise in view of our correspondence during the War. I began a period of three years of very exciting and interesting work. The experience of competent and effective anesthetic care for the sick, research into the unknown and the education of bright young people became an attractive change for me. My clinical experience in the Army during the war was great, but I really enjoyed much more, the academic Medical Center and its opportunities.

Just before my return, Rovenstine had put together the first Post Graduate Assembly in Anesthesiology in New York in the winter of 1945. It was designed to provide a high level refresher opportunity for returning veterans. The program was crafted by Rovey to consist of panel presentations of the major cutting edge of science for which clinical application was possible or had happened. This meeting was a great success and although there was a hiatus of one year before the next Assembly, it has grown annually to become one of the most important meetings in the Western world in anesthesiology. It now approaches its fiftieth anniversary in December of 1996. I was one of several people who helped Rovey put together the second Post Graduate Assembly in 1947 and then was of aid to Lewis Wright in his turn as General Chairman in organizing the next two Assemblies. My own turn, officially of three years, as the General Chairman and therefore constructor of the Assembly followed the work of Lewis Wright. I attended this fabulous meeting for twenty three consecutive years before moving to Miami as Dean of the Faculty of Medicine in 1969. Therefore an important part of my professional life, as far as scientific conventions were concerned, revolved around the planning, the maintenance and the enjoyment of this great anesthesiology Assembly that was begun by Rovey in 1945.

Those three post war years with him were stunning in their pleasure for me in many ways. I was by this time his first assistant in every respect in the New York University department. It was a great privilege for me to be the number two person. In return for much that I learned I worked as hard as I knew how to make this period a happy and productive one for both of us. Scientific research thrived. The relationships with the Department of Physiology and its outstanding faculty were resumed. Clinical care blossomed. There was an influx of very bright, capable young people who made it a great pleasure to teach such eager and attractive individuals. Among the many veterans of the war who were interested in anesthesiology and came to Rovey's Department were Richard Ament, Sam Denson and James West. They were prototypic of young physicians who had learned some anesthesia during the war and had been productive after initial rapid and quick immersion in "on the job" education in responsibilities to which they were assigned during the war. It was a great delight to see them at New York University getting what I think was the best education then available with all of its strong aspects restored and its advances appropriate to the newer developments that came from the war and from civilian life. Especially good for me was the fact that some of the people who had come to Bellevue to learn anesthesiology in the Rovenstine tradition were men with whom I had served and gotten started in anesthesiology. Denson and West were two of those who came to New York for their formal post war education.

The residency was a thrilling one. It was very strong educationally with the Monday night sessions, if anything, more powerful and more attractive than before the war and the clinical services extremely good with bright young anesthesiologists and equally bright and competent young surgeons also returning from the war to become civilians Once again.

In addition to being Rovey's number two person with all that implied, I had responsibilities as his junior partner in the private practice of anesthesiology including surgical anesthesia and diagnostic and therapeutic nerve block. He had a good private practice because of his very strong reputation with a good many distinguished surgeons, a number of whom had returned from senior positions in the Armed Forces during the war. As time went on, I often was invited or assigned to take care of some these patients. Over the three year period I began to develop a practice of my own that consisted of a modest number of wealthy patients undergoing straightforward operations and a larger number of patients who were very sick. The latter often had no money, or their insurance had been spent. It was something like Bellevue without tears. Most of these private practice patients were cared for either at the Doctor's Hospital in New York or at the New York Hospital, where I was always warmly welcomed by good friends, Donald Burdick at the Doctor's Hospital and Joseph Artusio at the New York Hospital. With Rovenstine's help and sponsorship I became reasonably well established in part-time private practice as well as in the academic world of anesthesiology at Bellevue.

It was clear to me from discussions with Rovey that although the time was not close, he was concerned about the succession of the Chairmanship at Bellevue. He wanted me to succeed him. He made it perfectly plain that that was his wish and we had a number of cordial conversations about it. It was flattering to me — but it was at least 15 years in the future because of Rovey's relative youth.

The arithmetic didn't suit me because the Bellevue Chair was too remote and vague for my future. I had definitely decided to prepare myself for an earlier opportunity to secure a Chair if one became available. But I think he understood it since it would make little sense for me to be waiting in the wings for fifteen years or more before having the opportunity I sought.

We had some discussion about my future from time to time. Our relationship continued to be a strong one professionally and personally and I believed he would want me to accept a Chair elsewhere if it was a very good opportunity. Shortly thereafter a great opportunity did come my way almost by chance. Elsewhere I have discussed the notion of opportunity of chance and the importance of grasping of it when it becomes available. This one concerns the situation at the College of Physicians and Surgeons of Columbia University and the Columbia-Presbyterian Medical Center.

A new Chairman of the Department of Surgery at Columbia had been appointed in 1946 upon Dr. Whipple's retirement as the Valentine Mott Professor of Surgery. He was a person who was going to figure in a very important way in my life in the future. His name was George H. Humphreys II. The Chairperson of the division of Anesthesiology in the Department of Surgery was the distinguished anesthesiologist, Virginia Apgar who was also one of my very good friends in New York City. Virginia Apgar was an extraordinary individual and her name is well known throughout the world of anesthesiology, pediatrics and the medical community because of her important contributions to neo-natal physiology, clinical care of the newborn and the Apgar Score, named for her.

After graduation from college at Mount Holyoke, Dr. Apgar came to Columbia's College of Physicians and Surgeons as one of the small number of women entering the profession in the early 1930's. She graduated from P&S with distinction. She wanted to be a surgeon but the then Chairman of Surgery, Dr. Allan O. Whipple, thought that the new field of anesthesiology would be an important one for her to learn and lead at the Presbyterian Hospital and at Columbia University.

One must recall the environment of the times. Dr. Whipple, understandably viewed anesthesiology as one of the branches of surgery, a view which was commonplace in his day. He wanted Dr. Apgar to be very well educated in this field and he knew about the Wisconsin school led by Waters and extended by Rovenstine to New York City. Accordingly, Dr. Apgar followed Dr. Whipple's "suggestion" and went to the University of Wisconsin where she spent a year with Dr. Waters and then returned to New York to work with Rovenstine at Bellevue. She then returned to the Presbyterian Hospital to lead the division of anesthesiology in the Department of Surgery. All went very well clinically. She established an anesthesia residency and built a moderate-sized attending staff for clinical anesthesiology with people who were very competent clinicians.

When Dr. Whipple retired and Dr. Humphreys assumed the Valentine Mott Chair in Surgery, it was his view and that of some of his colleagues, that a strong academic and research presence should be developed in anesthesiology in addition to its competent clinical service. This certainly was a far sighted view for the time [but understandable if one takes into account Dr. Humphreys' desire to have this additional capability to buttress the development of anesthesiology and surgery]. Also, it was a part of his character to improve all his divisions in surgery. Partly, also, because he was a thoracic and cardiac surgeon whose work was very dependent upon competent anesthesia and the development of newer knowledge in that field, he decided to do all he could to improve its academic productivity.

There were discussions with a few people, and I was one of them, about adding a research presence. I felt however that the situation was not a good one for Dr. Apgar nor for me in the way it was, at first, envisioned. My attitude, of course, was conditioned by Rovenstine's and Waters' points of view. Essentially their view was that an anesthesiology department of modern vintage (the end of the 1940s) should be independent in the Faculty of Medicine and that it should have research, clinical care and education of equal strength on a par with other departments in the Faculty of Medicine. This idea was not a common one by a long way but it seemed to sit well with George Humphreys and with his colleagues, but they were rightfully concerned about Virginia Apgar's views. They wanted to please her because she was so able a clinician and educator. It was important to make her happy and that was crucial to Humphreys and his colleagues.

She did not wish to be the Chairperson in the new structure for anesthesiology but she had great loyalty to Columbia and to the Presbyterian Hospital. She recommended to Dr. Humphreys that Bob Dripps and I were the best people to fill the role. She also agreed that she would be happy to stay on if either of us were appointed Chairman. My knowledge of the next series of events was made comfortable for me because of my excellent friendship with Virginia Apgar and my rapidly forming friendship with George Humphreys.

One must keep in mind the ambiance of the time in order to avoid misunderstanding the events that were proceeding. Some of them would be unthinkable problems today and others would be well understood. The environment was very specific. George Humphreys was recruiting a person to head the Division of Anesthesiology which was viewed by him and all of his colleagues as a part of his Department of Surgery. For that reason, unless he chose to, he did not have to have a search committee nor did he have to consult with the authorities in either the College of Physicians and Surgeons or the Presbyterian Hospital beyond what would normally be required by the addition of a person senior in rank in any academic department. In short he was not choosing a department chairman but a person whose work was viewed by most people at that time as a normal part of the surgical experience.

Dr. Robert Dripps of the University of Pennsylvania had several conversations with Drs. Apgar and Humphreys. He indicated quite clearly that he was not interested in leaving Philadelphia or the University of Pennsylvania and recommended me strongly as qualified to carry out the missions that they were contemplating at Columbia. I then had a series of discussions with George about the possibility of my carrying out his plans. These discussions took place beginning in the fall of 1948 and continued through the winter into the spring of 1949. I felt that it was absolutely necessary, despite my great happiness and desire to go to Columbia, an opportunity I never expected, to persuade George Humphreys and his colleagues in surgery and then other members of the faculty at Columbia that anesthesiology was not a part of surgery and that it needed to be an independent department in order to achieve its maximum potential for growth and development. In fact to achieve those goals that Humphreys and his colleagues wished to see accomplished would only be possible with an independent Department of Anesthesiology.

It was very difficult both intellectually and emotionally for me to institute the self-discipline not to eopardize the great joy of being invited to so distinguished an institution under the most favorable of conditions while feeling that it was essential to have an independent department like Rovenstine's, modeled on the one that was established by his mentor and teacher Ralph Waters at Wisconsin. I did not appreciate the problems I was presenting to George Humphreys since, at the time of these discussions, there were only two independent departments of anesthesiology in academic centers in the United States, the first being at Wisconsin and the second at New York University. In the Western world there was only one other independent department and that was at Oxford under the direction of Sir Robert Macintosh. Fortunately for me and for what this arrangement implied in connection with the development of anesthesiology, I proceeded as tactfully as possible and freely quoted the advice of Waters and Rovenstine who were respected at Columbia. It seemed to me that if the best way to accomplish Humphreys' mission was identical with my purposes and fully acceptable to Virginia Apgar that we must go in this direction. Happily for me personally in a very important way and I think of importance to the development of our field in the academic world, George

Humphreys was willing to accept my recommendation that an independent department be established by the Board of Trustees at Columbia University and an independent service at the Presbyterian Hospital within a period of three years. So important did I deem this process that I volunteered to leave if what I was going to bring to the medical center did not accomplish to their full satisfaction all that we were planning. Furthermore, I agreed that the Faculty and the Executive officers at the medical school and the hospital were to be the sole judges. Their decision would be final. I didn't realize how brash a condition this was. At the age of thirty four, there was little that didn't seem possible to achieve and much to my delight these suggestions, as I prefer to call them, rather than conditions of employment, were accepted by the various authorities and an independent department in the Faculty of Medicine at Columbia was established short of the three year proposal initially made. An independent service at the Presbyterian Hospital for anesthesiology was established simultaneously. I was appointed the Chairman of the University Department and the Director of the Clinical Service on New Year's Day of 1952.

It might be of interest to point out that these were not theoretical considerations brought to Dr., Humphreys' attention for his decision but were realities that made sense to him and which I thought essential to my growth and development and that of the projected department. For instance, I pointed out to him that there was very little that one could do in professional as well as interpersonal relationships with the members of the other six departments of surgery if they viewed me, understandably so, as a member of George Humphreys' department rather than as a colleague of independent status and equality with them. Some of them in fact told me that they were uncomfortable with my being in the Department of Surgery since they felt that they didn't have equal access to me or to my colleagues in terms of service to them. Also there could be a problem for me in doing collaborative educational or research work with other surgeons and members of the Departments of Medicine and Pediatrics as well.

Much to my delight George Humphreys saw that all of these connections needed to be made and was very supportive of the projected change if I "cut the mustard correctly." Therefore by the late spring of 1949 all the arrangements were put into place and I was invited to join the Columbia-Presbyterian Medical Center effective the 1st of July, 1949.

It was at this point that I began my discussions to obtain Dr. Rovenstine's concurrence and his advice about what to do about the appointment I was offered. He accepted the fact that I would leave and was pleased and proud that I would be going to an institution of world class rank to bring the Waters-Rovenstine philosophy to an enlarged platform in academic medicine. His advice was very helpful and warmly and freely given. There were some interesting status aspects of the transition period. George Humphreys felt that as an Assistant Professor at New York University it was somewhat inappropriate for me to stay at that rank with the prospect of being appointed a full Professor and ultimately a departmental chairman if all went well at Columbia. Rovenstine was most cooperative with that thought and I was promoted rapidly to the rank of Associate Professor of Anesthesiology at New York University so that the gap between Assistant Professor and Professor would be closed by the summer of 1949.

I could not come to Columbia on the 1st of July because Rovenstine had a major commitment to be part of an important teaching group in Europe. He was going to bring the principal achievements of American Anesthesiology to various centers in post war Europe along with a group of distinguished surgeons. All of this was to take place in the summer of 1949. I asked the Columbia people to agree to delay my arrival until right after Labor Day. They were somewhat disappointed at the delay after all the agreements were in place but they were very understanding and tolerant of my desire to fulfill my responsibility to Rovenstine and to New York University. In fact it would be helpful training for me to run that department on my own as preparation for going to the Columbia-Presbyterian Medical Center.

Rovenstine went on his mission to Europe and enjoyed it enormously and contributed a great deal to the tour.

On September 6, 1949 I moved to the Columbia-Presbyterian Medical Center. The Faculty of Medicine approved George Humphreys' recommendation that Virginia Apgar and I both be appointed full professors of anesthesiology. The Faculty approved her nomination prior to mine, which was a splrndid thing for them to do, as it gave her the status of being the first appointed Full Professor of Anesthesiology at Columbia University. She was the first woman to hold that rank at Columbia.

Virginia then went on richly earned and deserved sabbatical leave and returned in due course the following year when the next steps for the growth and development of her own career were destined to take place.

So many important things seem to happen by chance and yet, chance and opportunity are often missed by many of us. Chance was seen and seized by us when Virginia Apgar returned from her sabbatical leave. Some of this story goes back to a meeting that I had in Washington D.C. with Dr. Joseph Kreiselman who was a good friend of Dr. Rovenstine. The story bears some telling because of the hand of fate in a forecast that could not have been made at the time it occurred.

After the war in Europe ended, I had returned to Washington, D.C. to function as Chairman of the Section on Anesthesiology in the operating room of the Army's distinguished Walter Reed Hospital in the nation's capital. I had other duties for the Army which involved some work at the Pentagon as well. I had already made tentative arrangements to return to Dr. Rovenstine's department by then or at least the preliminary discussions were completed. I was in constant touch with Rovey during that period and he urged me to call upon his good friend Joe Kreiselman who was one of the highly respected and senior people in the anesthesiology world of Washington D.C. Joe's specialty was obstetrical anesthesia and he was extraordinarily competent and versatile in this field. He developed apparatus that was suitable for the resuscitation of the newborn and other apparatus for the treatment of both mother and child with care and with sensitivity at a time when very few people were paying much attention to anesthesia for obstetrics. The parturient was not viewed as someone who required very good medical care but as a person needing help in supplementing nature's way of doing whatever was required.

Accordingly I called Dr. Kreiselman and made an appointment to see him. He was very kind and invited me to a family dinner at his beautiful home. This was the first time I had met a great man in our field face to face in an orbit that was not directly Dr. Rovenstine's yet was due to his making the arrangements. I thought I was going to be making a simple courtesy call and found that I was completely enchanted by this very bright and able individual who was so dedicated to making obstetrical anesthesia and the peri-natal period a safer and happier experience for both mother and child. I was starry-eyed by his enthusiasm and by his desire to make obstetrical patients the object of attention by the best minds in clinical medicine. He also felt that newborn research which was very scarce in the traditional sense except for the development of small pieces of apparatus needed to be sponsored and done. In the course of one conversation he looked at me intensely and said: "I hope that what I am telling you will make an impression upon you ." Well it certainly did. He then asked me to promise him that *when* I became a departmental chairman in an area of influence in anesthesiology I would set up a strong obstetrical anesthesia service and develop peri-natal anesthesia in collaboration among the three groups that were necessary, i.e. obstetrics, pediatrics and anesthesiology. I thought he was a bit over enthusiastic and perhaps had had one glass of wine too many but I certainly did not think that I would be in any position to activate any of the ideas that I had heard from him or to devote a serious effort in that direction. However I was young and impressionable and convinced and I hastily and perhaps conveniently promised him that I would do what he asked.

When my appointment to Columbia was announced I received a call from Joe Kreiselman. He said: "I want to remind you of your promise. Please do something soon about obstetrics and perinatal care and all the things we talked about in Washington.." What a memory! I asked Dr. Apgar if it was a worthy use of her time to put an obstetrical and neonatal group together. She happily volunteered to do so and of course the rest is history. The first major effort in peri-natal care among the three disciplines was achieved at Columbia. I viewed myself as the message carrier and did all I could to support Virginia's efforts. Howard Taylor in Obstetrics and Gynecology and Rustin McIntosh in Pediatrics were most cooperative. Both were very cooperative in approving our bringing Stanley James to Virginia's unit and setting up a major research program among the three departments, designed by Apgar, James and their colleagues. Virginia Apgar's contributions to this field were outstanding. They were major and magnificent including the highly regarded and universally used Apgar score to evaluate the new born. Stanley James brought a distinguished research presence to the program.

After setting those important matters in place following my arrival at the Columbia-Presbyterian Medical Center I felt it would be very useful to visit all of the people who were in the several departments at this great medical center and to follow the example of both Waters and Rovenstine by doing what I could to understand the clinical service, its requirements and the principle of providing the best possible anesthetic care to patients by making this the first priority. I called on various key senior surgeons in the various departments of surgery to tell them of my keen interest in making things as good as possible for them and to remind them that we already had in place a residency program of modest size and a number of very able clinicians on the attending staff. I also wanted to be sure to indicate to those splendid anesthesiologists who were very good at clinical care that my purpose was to support and strengthen them in view of their crucial contributions to a department which was going to be changing direction but would never abandon or modify the concentration on superb clinical care. I think these efforts seemed valuable and agreeable to most of them.

To aid further in my gaining understanding of the people as well as the needs of our institution I also made myself available every night and weekend to give any attending surgeon who wished, the opportunity to call me into the hospital to work with him and give anesthesia to his patients. This offer was taken up with frequency. Whatever the reason, I spent a lot of nights and weekends for the first several years in operating rooms and therefore got to know almost all of the senior surgeons and a goodly number of the junior surgeons by so doing. My view about learning about the resident staff was also to spend a good deal of useful time being with them. I presided over all of the staff conferences which were frankly and advantageously modeled upon Rovenstine's Monday night Classical staff conference. In the early phases ours were not as good as his by far but the model was salutary and evolution took place rather rapidly as the teaching program was put into place and as the caliber of residents improved in a relatively short time. These conferences became major attractions to the anesthesia community in the greater New York area.

The conferences were recorded on reels and provide a fascinating record of lectures by this country's and the world's most distinguished anesthesiologists [in addition to valuable talks given by all of us in the Columbia Department of Anesthesiology. Other outstanding anesthesiologists, clinicians and scientists also spoke]. The reels were converted to 380 cassettes by Audio-Digest at the request of Mr. Patrick Sim, director of the Wood Library-Museum of Anesthesiology. These tapes are now a resource for all anesthesiologists, thanks to Mr. Sim, the Wood Library-Museum and its Board of Trustees and Audio Digest who did it pro bono.

I also had breakfast most mornings between 6:00 a.m. and 6:30 a.m. with the residents who were on call the night before. I valued the experience a great deal and I think most of the residents did so too. We got to know each other very much better and much more quickly so that I knew what needed to be done to improve their opportunities and they knew pretty much what to expect of their new leader and teacher. We talked at these breakfasts and we also saw patients about whom the residents were concerned. I should state that this was a period when attending anesthesiologists took their night and weekend call from home instead of being in the hospital physically. Therefore residents willy-nilly, were both saddled with and given the opportunity of fairly independent action since geographical distancing made immediate responsiveness by the faculty on call impossible. I worried about this situation for a good many years but learned to accept it since I could not improve upon it in our evolving specialty where the sensitivity of underpaid faculty members was beginning to have important repercussions.

It was easier and better to engage in private practice at much larger incomes and with very few onerous duties. On the useful side to us, it sorted out the individuals who were dedicated to an academic career for intellectual or other valid purposes. There was unfortunately and perhaps necessarily a good deal of moonlighting by these highly competent attending anesthesiologists because their incomes from the Presbyterian Hospital who paid all of us were simply unreasonably low. These had to be supplemented if they were to take care of their families and their children in the ways that had meaning for them. I have always regretted the fact that more could not be done for them financially. Their devotion to the academic purpose could not only have been purer in concept but more effective in aiding them to achieve goals which conformed as closely as possibly to their native talents. One wonders, even now, why a wealthy hospital with no restraints on charges behaved so poorly to a gifted staff of attending anesthesiologists with respect to their well earned compensation. It is not enough to say that everybody in the academic world did it. We should have been different.

The financial arrangements, such as they were, are something of a reminder of what goes on in professional athletics today. Great athletes like Babe Ruth in baseball, Sid Luckman in football and others of this caliber experienced in their time, despite their vast talents, a gross underpayment for their needs and for their abilities. As Stan Musial, one of the baseball greats put it, "In my day we were grossly underpaid and today's athletes are equally and vastly overpaid." I think it is fair to state that the analogy, while imperfect, was quite close to the mark in that very talented people in anesthesiology in full time careers in the academic health centers were insignificantly paid compared to their colleagues in private practice. The discrepancy in the earliest years of the middle part of the Twentieth Century was gross and unreasonable. I think it is also fair to say that anesthesiologists in later years were overpaid in the private practice sector as were physicians in many other specialties where physical action was the watchword.

These problems came under some kind of control in the mid to late 60's, probably expedited by the enactment of the Medicare amendments to Social Security. At that time academic physicians, including anesthesiologists, were able to bill for their services in the same way as others did and it narrowed the gap between those in private practice and those who wished to do full time work in the academic environment. Often payment was too generous to both groups for the welfare of the paying public to absorb. We are now, unfortunately, in another period of overcorrection by managed care.

There were other problems that a thirty-four year old head of anesthesiology services needed to learn to solve. Although my education in science and in clinical practice and especially in those intangible and very important areas that I learned from Dr. Rovenstine was excellent, I was not familiar with other kinds of information that were essential if one was to develop an outstanding multifaceted department at the Columbia-Presbyterian Medical Center. How was I to learn about the world of anesthesiology around me?

In 1950 I had the very great pleasure of participating in the care of a patient who was destined to become one of my very good friends and a diligent and outstanding supporter of my work and that of my colleagues. This was Mr. Charles B. Wrightsman about whom much more will be mentioned later on in this book. However, relevant to this particular problem to be solved, Charles urged that I should visit the very best places in anesthesiology in the United States and if possible in Western Europe. He promised that he would fund and take care of all the expenses I incurred in so doing. His suggestion was a very novel idea to me and I proceeded to think about which institutions to visit and how to make as few mistakes as possible in the selection of those institutions. Naturally I went back to Rovey and also discussed these questions with my very close friend Bob Dripps at the University of Pennsylvania and several other people as well. I came up with a modest list of institutions to visit in the United States and in the United Kingdom.

Anesthesia in the United Kingdom was very well developed at that time compared to the rest of continental Europe and other parts of the world. The great development on the continent was yet to come following the establishment of the Center for Academic Training and Advancement in Anesthesiology in Copenhagen right after the war under the direction of the distinguished professor of surgery at the University of Copenhagen, Professor Erik Husfeldt. Also there was enormous progress in America after the return of World War II veterans to institutions in the United States. It will be of interest to describe a a few of these visits to illustrate the kind of knowledge and information that I was to obtain that would help to infuse energy, talent and progress in the soon to be created department of anesthesiology at Columbia University and the independent anesthesiology service in the Presbyterian Hospital.

One of my visits was to the Massachusetts General Hospital's Anesthesia Service under the direction of Dr. Henry K. Beecher. Beecher was very well known at the time for his distinguished study of pain during the Italian campaign in World War II. It led to remarkable studies not only during the war but after it on methods of securing pain relief and improved understanding of the placebo factorr. People he collected around him in the pain studies included such very able people as Arthur Keats, Louis Lasagna and in intensive care Henning Pontoppidan and others.

Dr. Beecher was very kind and considerate to me. He spent a great deal of time showing me the clinical, educational and research activities of his splendid department. I was also impressed by the galaxy of stars from Europe who spent some time at the Massachusetts General Hospita, including Erik Nielson and Dick Thompson of Lund in Sweden and Bjorn Ibsen of Copenhagen in Denmark.

Beecher and I had lively discussions about many subjects. One of them was the value of nurse anesthetists in an academic department. Nurse anesthesia was, and is, a common feature of many strong anesthesia services in the academic and private practice worlds. While respecting his (and others) views of this subject, I felt it would be better to have a pure Wisconsin type group of only physicians administering anesthesia at the Columbia-Presbyterian Medical Center. That subject is still controversial. It seems, in 1996, that the importance of cost controls will have a strong voice in settling the debate. My earliest decision in 1950 was for an all physician department but that seems to have given way to a mixed group of physicians and nurses almost everywhere in America in 1996.

The research work performed under Beecher's leadership was brilliant, conceptually very strong and its applications to clinical problems were both large and important. I learned the importance of monitoring of respiratory function, of metabolic activity during anesthesia, of new approaches to pain therapy, of ethics in carrying out experiments on human subjects and the importance of the placebo effect. These very great gains in one department made me wish to have a large capability in a diverse number of special fields in anesthesiology. We would then be in a position to provide leadership to the field which was destined to find its way into the various sub-specialties. I was convinced that when enough knowledge had been gathered by research, it was necessary to effect clinical application as soon as possible

Subspecialization would be needed because the generalist in anesthesia could no longer be expert in everything. We would have to subspecialize to be really good.

One of the visits to departments from which I expected to learn important things to bring back to the development of the Columbia-Presbyterian department of anesthesiology was to the superb program at the University of Pennsylvania headed by Dr. Robert D. Dripps. This first visit gave me the opportunity of observing their clinical practice, their research activities and their educational programs in considerable detail. Clinical care of patients was outstanding and also served as a practical teaching forum for the residents and the fellows of that department. I made pre and post operative rounds with the senior surgeons as well as with the anesthesiologists and learned how oriented they were to personal relationships with patients. This needed to be developed and preserved at home as an item of first priority. The research effort was extraordinarily well balanced between basic science motivated by the desire to understand "nature" as applied to anesthesiology and the application of that research knowledge to clinical care. The educational program was incredibly strong in all its forms. The department was particularly gifted in having a large number of very effective lecturers and seminar teachers.

The important presence of Dr. Julius Comroe of Pennsylvania's Graduate School was a strong influence on the Department of Anesthesiology both as to the substance of research and its brilliant exposition in teaching. The faculty included, in addition to Dr. Dripps, a most distinguished leader of the group, such outstanding experts as James Eckenhoff, Leroy Vandam, Austin Lamont and a succession of highly competent younger people who followed in their footsteps. Because of the excellence of this department and the many things to learn from it and because of my now strongly developed close personal friendship with Bob Dripps, my visits to the Pennsylvania department and stays with Bob and Diana Dripps at their beautiful home became frequent. I was in Philadelphia approximately every six weeks to two months for a period of a several years. We enjoyed very happy and productive conversations and the most friendly of debates, incisive as well as warm in a personal sense. Although Bob Dripps was thought by many people who worked with or near him to be extraordinarily capable, few people seem to have seen the warmth of his spirit and the outstanding friendliness of his personality, particularly for someone with so competitive a professional nature as he had, competitive in the best sense of that word. He was educating and preparing me to challenge him and his institution for the premier reputation as "the best" of our field. He gave of himself unstintingly knowing that this was part of what I was there for. He was of immeasurable help in pursuing that goal and our friendship warmed and flourished until his untimely death in 1973. So close was our relationship that the family asked me to speak at his funeral and to deliver the eulogy on their behalf. His death was a monumental loss to me personally and also professionally, and a gigantic loss to our field.

Another visit of great interest for me was to the Mayo Clinic. My goal was to examine at close range the very important research work that was being done by Dr. Albert Faulconer on the correlation of EEG activity with the measured concentration of anesthetic agents in the blood. He was studying quantitatively the depth of anesthesia with a target (EEG) indicator. It was deemed highly desirable to objectively quantify the depth of anesthesia for better care of patients as well as to compare newer anesthetic agents with old ones. Faulconer and his colleagues were using the electro-encephalographic knowledge developed at the Mayo Clinic department of neurology and making correlations with an acoustic analyzer in the experiments with diethyl ether. It was very rewarding to learn from Albert about the various aspects of his research including the high technology, the brilliant strategies of investigation, and very astute design of the experiments for the purposes at hand. We also had considerable opportunity to talk about research and education in anesthesiology and I learned much from his very capable views of what the future might look like in both these areas. He was later to have the opportunity when he became Chairman of the Mayo department to put into operation many ideas which brought his department to a new height of excellence.

However Rochester, Minnesota is not exactly a metropolis. There are interesting customs that deal with the Mayo Clinic staff and its own rather closely bound group, all dedicated to the performance of outstanding clinical services because all of their patients had to come from somewhere else for the expert care they would get at the Mayo Clinic. I used that opportunity to learn something more about clinical care. I stayed at the Kahler Hotel which had all the facilities of a hospital room appropriate for the early 1950's. It was at first a bit startling to see a bedpan hung on the wall of a hotel room but one soon understood what the message was. I had heard from many of my friends who were patients at the Mayo Clinic how efficient and effective it was. I elected with Albert's help to have the experience of a patient during my visit and I actually went through the admissions process, the referral for laboratory data and the referral to specialists. I was amazed by how efficient, friendly and compassionate their system was in seeing that patients were well cared for in every respect. It was very simple and easy and there was no waiting on going from place to place in the system. The entire work-up was done briskly, with tenderness and with great medical expertise. It was a very important experience in learning about efficient and effective care of patients.

However all of these excellent experiences are not the entire story of my visit. I had committed, as I was soon to learn, an important social blunder in my visit. At the time that I was at the Mayo Clinic the very highly regarded and powerful Dr. John S. Lundy was the Chairman of that department. He was an expert clinician and particularly strong in the performance of nerve blocks for surgical procedures. I had, unfortunately for me, not written to him prior to my visit nor asked for the privilege of watching him do various nerve block procedures for surgical operations. He was not only accustomed to an audience but very much expected it while he was working. He was considerably put out by what he deemed to be lack of proper recognition of his outstanding skills through my failure to ask to see him or to watch him work. The first inkling of trouble was when he told Albert that he hoped that *Albert's guest* would be available for dinner that evening at the dining room of the Mayo Clinic. It explained to me why Albert was popping pills, presumably anti-headache preparations, because he knew of the trouble that was coming while I in my naive and uninformed manner was totally oblivious to the near chaos and havoc that I had unintentionally wrought! I went to the dinner as expected and Dr. Lundy was caustic beyond belief both to me and to Albert. I learned much from this experience and was sorry that I had given my good friend Albert Faulconer so much trouble, albeit unwittingly.

Needless to say I learned much about academic monarchs who did not require actual thrones or kingly regalia to make known their strong position of autocratic control. Over the nearly half century since that visit I probably learned almost as much about how to treat the "star" and academic tyrant as about anesthesiology and its efforts to improve patient care, education and to enlarge the scope of research.

In the United Kingdom, I visited several of the teaching hospitals in London and the very strong department under the leadership of Professor William Mushin in the Welsh National School of Medicine in Cardiff, Wales. I also visited outside of London the University of Liverpool directed by the highly competent Professor T. Cecil Gray. In London I spent most of my time at the Westminster Hospital whose anesthesia consultant group was chaired by Professor Geoffrey Organe, soon to be knighted for his extraordinary accomplishments in leading his department to a major influence upon the development of British anesthesia in the young National Health Service of the United Kingdom. The future Sir Geoffrey Organe also had associates of considerable talent in his service. The striking thing to me was the differences in attitude of the British from the American surgeons in the way operating room activity was conducted.

Surgical operation proceeded at a very fast pace compared to that in the United States and very skillfully. British anesthesia therefore had to accommodate to a very different kind of surgical tempo and did so with good sense and alacrity. The British anaesthetists in those days did less monitoring of vital signs than was customary in the United States. They argued that the speed and quality of their surgical operations were such as to not require any closer observation. The British also were pioneering in the use of muscle relaxants and the newest of the inhalant anesthetic agents, halothane. The skills exercised in the Westminster Hospital were very strong indeed and I was puzzled as to what I could bring back to New York from these experiences to accommodate to the realities of surgical practices.

At St. Thomas' Hospital in London I was struck also by the very great skill of both surgeons and anesthesiologists and of the vast intelligence of many of the members of the staff who were consultants in the new National Health Service. I was particularly impressed by the late Dr. Harry Churchill-Davidson and by Dr. Derek Wylie. A major activity undertaken by these two very able British anaesthetists was the writing of their superb textbook, superior to anything that had previously been written and destined to become the standard aanesthesia text for a good many years to come. It was strong evidence of a powerful interest in education new to our field. Their book was literate, complete and extremely easy to use in the education of the British registrar and the American resident.

In Wales, Professor Mushin had also developed a very strong group in patient care and education. The research that he and his colleagues conducted was extremely important and it was conditioned by Professor Mushin's strong interest in respiration. He and Dr. Rendell-Baker made outstnadingly valuable contributions to the development of apparatus designed to provide automatic ventilation of the lungs in a physiological manner. As time went on and the young people became seasoned, their research interest broadened and extended to clinical pharmacology, the management of pain, obstetrical anesthesia and other fields. Michael Rosen was one of those preparing to be leaders in education, organizational matters and in research.

The department in Wales also typified the importance of interest on the part of government and the people in the immediate post World War II period in the development of anesthesia. The reason that Mushin went from Oxford, where he was Professor Sir Robert McIntosh's assistant, to Wales was the observation by the coroner's office that mortality due to anesthesia in Cardiff was so severe and serious in 1946 that something had to be done about it. The answer fortunately for Welsh and worldwide medicine was the invitation to Mushin to come and set things right in Wales. He proceeded to do this with astonishing vigor and with outstanding results [in improving the anesthetic care of patients] in Cardiff. This influence, of course, spread to the rest of the United Kingdom and to all parts of the world where the need for safe and competent anesthesia was realized.

The story in Liverpool was a somewhat different one. I looked forward to meeting Professor Gray because he was the person who crafted and popularized the use of general anesthesia with nitrous oxide and oxygen and muscle relaxants. My visit to Professor Gray's department was a great revelation in many respects. I saw how effectively they were able to use the combination of light general anesthesia with nitrous oxide and oxygen supplemented with narcotics when needed and with muscle relaxants. Patients did well, the surgical field was fine, and the patients were restored to consciousness with very great ease and rather quickly. Gray was also a charismatic leader and an excellent clinician as well as a very competent educator in the strong traditions of British lecture and seminar activity. The research in the department was designed to bring quick applications to clinical problems.

Dr. Jackson Rees was one of the important figures in pediatric anesthesia in Liverpool. Jackson Rees was also an extremely competent figure and had done almost miraculous work in practical research as well as clinical anesthesia care children, taking into account their various physiological differences from adults at a time when this was not commonly done. He developed new apparatus to deliver the fruits of the newer knowledge of the anesthesia needs of infants and children.

I was extraordinarily well treated in every respect and the friendships I formed with these two individuals and some members of their department [were long lasting and] have continued to this day. The visit was also marked by my first experience with the lack of central heating in mid twentieth century during the British winter. I remember with great concern which way one should face the roaring fire. Facing it head on meant a very cold back side and in reverse it was a freezing nose with the symptoms of coryza! It was also a novel experience for me to be led to my bedroom in the Gray household with heated bricks to keep my feet warm!

Finally in the United Kingdom there was my great visit to the Nuffield Department at Oxford under the distinguished leadership of Sir Robert McIntosh. Mac, as everyone called him, was a very great friend of Rovenstine's. They had an uncommonly close relationship and respect for each other and some of this rubbed off on me. Sir Robert viewed me as one of Rovey's students who was in the process of trying to develop and make a mark for himself in his new institution. Clinical anesthetic care at the Radcliffe Infirmary, the clinical venue for anesthesia and surgery at Oxford was very good and very strong. Sir Robert was one of the world's most gifted leaders of anesthesia t and his influence was clearly felt everywhere. His research was intended to design apparatus that could be used in third world countries under primitive conditions. Mr. Salt, the superb technician in the Oxford department, helped build the various pieces of equipment that the Professor wished to use for these purposes. Over time many outstanding individuals were attracted to the department at Oxford. Among them were, in addition to Mushin, Pask, Nunn and Prys-Roberts — all destined to assume leadership roles in British Anaesthesia.

My experiences in the United Kingdom gave me much to bring back to Columbia and the Presbyterian Hospital but they would have to be shaped and crafted somewhat differently. The professorial unit was designed for the education of medical students, for research and for a specific type of education for registrars. The Professor had no greater jurisdiction over the clinical services in the institution than any other active consultant in the National Health Service. In the 1950's that particular model seemed unsuitable for transfer to the United States and to my own institution. The tradition in America and at the Columbia-Presbyterian Medical Center was too strong to change from having a single individual in charge of the academic activities of the department and director of the clinical service of a particular specialty. In my view the American system lent itself to more effective coordination of the two activities which, when all is said and done, should be mutually reinforcing rather than isolated. On the other hand should there be a change in either the availability of residents or in their attitudes toward their functions in a great medical center some change in the coordinated pattern might have to be considered. Such consideration may be useful for end of century anesthesiology in the United States.

At this writing, in 1996, a time for change in the residency program has indeed arrived. It is marked by a sharp reduction in the number of residents entering anesthesiology. Also, there seems to be in the minds of many a surplus of anesthesiologists. If that is so, then it makes more sense to regard the residency as an educational experience for smaller numbers, and training with the individual services as a cornerstone of education rather than of service to the institution. This might call for the kind of organization of clinical care and education that the British have used. Another difference that might be used constructively in New York would be to add the application of instrumentation, medical devices and other machinery to the intellectual aspects of research. In short, the Americans could profit by an increased sensitivity to research subserving patient care. Finally, the idea of a National Health Service as the backbone of the health care of the nation was a very appealing one as I saw it in operation. Obviously there were problems with this system [as with any other] and since they belong to the welfare state such a method of clinical care would meet even stronger resistance in the United States of today..

An anticipated outcome of the visits to the best American and British institutions was a sharpened focus on the goals for the department at the Columbia-Presbyterian Medical Center. I saw that first priority had to be the continued development of superb clinical care. We would have to plan for the same end result that one saw in Britain but with different strategies and techniques in order to accommodate to the longer duration of surgical procedures in the United States and New York area. It is not useful to discuss the reasons for these differences since [that tends to lead to unwarrented criticism and finger pointing. In any event] it is useless to attempt to change the pattern of surgery to accommodate to a fixed model of anesthesia. The intellectual attitudes of surgeons in the United Kingdom differ from those of the United States.

Nurses in anesthesia had no place in the United Kingdom apparently by law. Attitudes in the United States in the institutions I visited varied markedly. My own taste, in keeping with Waters' tradition, supported the idea that reliable patient care and individual attention to each patient is better served by a person trained in medicine who specializes in anesthesiology. This view is obviously a controversial one and, at the time of writing in 1996, is a cause of considerable heat and argument because of the pressures to control costs. The unexpected revelation that it is not less expensive to have nurses than physicians may in fact be the result of time constraints traditional in nursing care. Overtime pay for anesthetic nurses is often larger than for physicians and the costs are therefore greater. However, I decided that it would be feasible, to have an all physician department at the Columbia-Presbyterian Medical Center in 1950: the four nurse anesthetists who remained in the department on my arrival were properly and affectionately pensioned when they reached the age of retirement. Miss Anne Penland, a very important nurse anesthetist at the Presbyterian Hospital in an earlier part of the twentieth century, was still at the hospital at my arrival three decades later. She was a warmly welcoming person, very intelligent and of invaluable aid to me in trying to put into place our projected goals for patient care. I think of her as a major contributor to affairs at the Presbyterian Hospital and a major advisor to a young stranger trying to accomplish the missions that the majority of the faculty wished to see completed.

The trip to look at excellent departments in the United States and then in Britain had reaffirmed that expanded depth and breadth of very high quality patient care was the first priority of the department. Certain changes in organization were necessary. In addition to having talented and highly skillful individuals at all levels of the attending staff, residents and fellows, it also became apparent that a decentralized structure to serve specific functions in various environments would be necessary. Ed Hanks, as leader and manager, was the hero of our decentralized plan of organization.

It was highly desirable for anesthesiologists to become familiar with the problems of the various surgical services by close contact with the various surgeons in each specialty. The organization of the various departments of surgery made it possible to have such regular assignments of our staff. Another good byproduct of this arrangement was the close contact with other professional groups such as the nursing department in operating rooms and on the various surgical floors. However, identifying anesthesiologists who had the talent and the drive to implement these plans was difficult.

So important was that program that we aggresively educated people to fulfill the plan. Growth was not only vigorous, but extraordinarily rapid because there were no important barriers for intelligent people who wished to satisfy their ambitions. It was these kinds of people that I sought to attract or train. This meant bringing able people to our residency and research fellowship before they could be invited to learn how to lead our various to-be-created units.

At Columbia the time was as exciting as Camelot must have been in ancient Britain. The basic science departments were outstanding. There were no areas of weakness. The clinical departments were powerful, highly respected, and valued, and there was unlimited support for academic anesthesiology among a galaxy of stars. With the great help of important surgeons, in addition to Dr. Humphreys individuals like Fordyce B. St. John, Rudoph Schullinger, Robert (Pat) Elliott, Robert Wylie, Milton Porter, and Arthur Voorhees, as well as many others, the new discipline in the Medical Center was guaranteed strong support and was sure to thrive. Other collaborators in surgery like David Habif, Frank Stinchfield, and John Lattimer, were critically important to our development and our hopes for success. In medicine, the physicians Robert Loeb, Stanley Bradley, the then young resident and now highly distinguished leader at the Memorial Sloan-Kettering Institution, Paul Marx, and Noble Laureates Dickinson Richards, and Andre Cournand, were all there in support of anesthesiology, its leadership, and its evolving staff who were selected for their major potential in academic competence, as well as leadership for the future.

Things took on an aura of vast excitement, and there arose a strong feeling of family affection among its members, and of mutual support. It is hard to imagine today, but in the beginning of the 1950s clinical competence in anesthesiology of the sort that one now takes for granted in even the most modest of small community hospitals, was then only available in a few major academic institutions, of which Columbia was one. A relatively small number of us who had the clinical skills, took on willingly, and accepted happily, the burden of day and night work which was a major consumer of time, as well as energy, in order to establish the clinical credibility of anesthesiology. In the early years, for example, I did no official night call because I was on call *all the time,* and was always asked to give anesthesia by the senior surgeons, or physicians of the day who felt that the best anesthetic care then available in the institution was necessary for a given patient.

The work was hard but far from onerous. There was the happiness of being useful and constructive in the care of many people whose illnesses needed special skills that were unfortunately possessed by relatively small numbers of anesthesiologists. The education of residents was expanded more rapidly than previously, and the scientific growth of individuals vastly improved to conform to the same standards of excellence as other distinguished units at Columbia. The research program was begun with great difficulties considering the fact that there were few scientists, no resources, and no space available at the outset. These efforts were helped by the magnificent and major support of several grateful patients who learned about anesthesiology from their own or their family's experiences, and were most helpful in funding the earliest efforts at scientific research. It was only later on that major N.I.H. support for research became available.

There was, unusual for those days, also a required clinical clerkship in anesthesiology for all medical students at the College of Physicians and Surgeons. The educational program for the residents consisted in close teaching and supervision in the operating rooms, and also, participation in staff conferences in which the residents took a very active part.

The Columbia Department educated the majority of its graduates for clinical practice in anesthesiology as was common then, and is common today. However, a special interest that my colleagues and I had which we maintained always, was to develop leaders in anesthesiology as a deliberate and important part of faculty development. This is neither an arcane nor an esoteric subject because one of the crucial aspects of the development of any organization, institution, or field of endeavor is dependent upon the presence and availability of strong leadership. We decided to undertake consciously, and deliberately, the education for leadership in academic anesthesiology a few years after the end of World War II (1949). Our focus was to be on the development and education of potential department chairmen for the future, the encouragement of leadership in the research aspects of this field, and of course, the production of senior educators and clinicians as well.

The conscious effort resulted in the development of substantial numbers of future chairmen. The exact number is unknown to me but exceeds sixty. Good protoplasm, excellent instincts and careful nurturing were needed. It was nature *and* nurture.

One might ask why the Columbia-Presbyterian Medical Center would be willing to do these revolutionary things at that time! Not many institutions were equipped to discharge these functions. It was a youthful and joyous period and new leaders could begin their work relatively early in our evolution as a major force in American medicine. Furthermore, Columbia and its leadership enjoyed an environment that had almost everything. Osler described it (in another connection) this way "and binding us all together, there came as a sweet influence, the spirit of the place; teacher and taught alike, felt the presence and subtle domination of greatness, comradeship, and empathy with one another. Devotion to work, were its fruits and its guidance drove from each heart hatred and malice, and all uncharitable feelings."

How did we go about achieving the purpose so easy to set forth, and so difficult to accomplish? The proposal by John Gardner that leadership is a process of persuasion, and example by which an individual or a team induces a group to take action that is in accordance with the leader's purposes for the good of the organization, was our basic tenet. The idea that leaders are "born and not made" was rejected outright, while recognizing that qualities such as stamina, intellect, and others were part of an individual's makeup and necessary for leadership. The attitude was George Bernard Shaw 's when he said that it is stupid to say that a person of great talent is born and not made, *since all of us are born and not made.*

The plan therefore, was to try to identify young individuals who could think long-term, who had wide general interests, and who understood and valued vision and intangible qualities, individuals who could cope with conflict and had the ability to make prompt decisions, and equally important, who could think for themselves in terms of dynamic renewal, recognizing that both boredom and obsolescence were possible, unless there was renewal continually.

In addition, it was necessary to find individuals whose sense of competition, while keen, was so secure, that they would be able, and comfortable to surround themselves with highly competent people. Since their preparation was for leadership roles at other institutions, they had to have ability to understand new cultures, and to adapt to them quickly. They had to have communications skills, including literate writing, and excellent verbal skills. From an operational standpoint, to carry out this deliberate plan, the departmental Chairman had to have precise goals, and yet be flexible enough to meet unexpected opportunities.

How does one consciously try to develop leaders? Assuming native intelligence, talent, physical stamina, and the willingness to work hard, the prospective leader in training, needs to have opportunities and challenges which are not static, but grow with his ability to master the problems he encounters. This process involves structuring a department in such a way that there is considerable decentralization into small units if the department is large, and to use the same principle of control if the department is small. The prospective leader becomes, as part of his tuitional process, the leader of a small group, sometimes only two or three people at first. He is helped and encouraged, and has frequent private conversations with his Chairman to review his successes and triumphs, and to deal with the problems and the inevitable failures he encounters. To the extent that it is possible, a pattern of reassignment should occur, so that the future leader will have changing challenges and opportunities in a reasonable period of time, and that they will be enlarging ones.

In the education of a prospective leader, there is the absolute necessity to encourage reasonable risk taking, and to tolerate failure, so that the learning opportunity of dealing with the problems that failure brings, will be available to that prospective leader — obviously never at the expense of patient welfare or safety. He has to learn to speak well, therefore, he has to be given speaking opportunities in an ever escalating environment of difficulty from the most simple, to the most complex and critical audiences. He must learn to write in a style that is uniquely his, and yet with a clarity that guarantees self-improvement. He must meet new people and new cultures, and new environments. The sabbatical leave process is one way of doing this. His triumphs and successes must be praised quickly, and reinforced where justified, and his lack of success, providing it occurs as a result of prudent risk taking and not as a result of stupidity, must be tolerated and gently channeled back to the proper path. Like an outstanding tennis athlete, or perhaps a musician, he has to be able to concentrate on overcoming the errors of the past without undue self-mortification, and to look to the future for a new opportunity to do things better. The scholar of classical Greek Literature, E.L. Dodds, put it this way about another subject: "If truth is beyond our grasp, the errors of tomorrow are still to be preferred to the errors of today; for error in the sciences is only another name for the progressive approximation to truth."

Perhaps, the most difficult aspect of the preparation for leadership comes out of the realization that a departmental Chairman in anesthesiology is often chosen for his past accomplishments usually, in scientific research, rarely in education or patient care, and only occasionally for organization skills. Today business or economic abilities and business management skills are very much valued. The future leader must understand thoroughly that his next assignment, whatever else it may be, must include service to others, i.e., his followers; the willingness, and in fact, the desire to see that his new constituents have even greater opportunities than he had, and perhaps, most of all, to respect and to love young people whom he is privileged to lead in his new role. Finally, when his time comes to relinquish the leadership role, if his mental and physical agility permit, he should evolve further and accepti functions that produce little glory.

How conscious is the process of preparation for leadership? — and how much of just personal friendship associated with the "Old Boy" system is involved? The preparation *by* the leader is highly conscious. The trainee for leadership must be brought along slowly and monitored carefully, until the *idea* of leadership becomes his own. Eventually, friendship develops,. a feeling of close family ties and personal affection. However, feelings or emotions — even in "tranquillity contemplated" should not cloud judgment. Some of the most wonderful and delightful people do not become effective leaders, and this sad fact must be recognized and accepted.

Research at Columbia was also a major activity. Many of the faculty were engaged in large and complex problems, including some of the earliest of studies on pharmacokinetics, which consists of unraveling the influence of living organs, tissues and cells upon the disposition of anesthetic drugs and agents in the body. Also under investigation was the development of methods of improving clinical care, notably in the intensive care setting that especially concerned thoracic and cardiovascular surgical patients and pediatric patients. Respiration, circulation and renal and hepatic function as influenced by anesthetic agents were also studied. A major research program was pursued in obstetrical anesthesia and the physiology of the newborn.

As in the Waters tradition, research competence had to be redeveloped as a serious venture for talented individuals. They needed to learn from highly competent basic scientists. There is really no short cut to learning about research, and at the times when I decided on the direction we would go it required a number of matters to fall into place. It required among other things picking people with a serious interest in research and finding a place for them and people to teach them in a happy but uncompromising environment with respect to skills. I felt very strongly that our department in 1950 did not have the requisite credentials to educate scientists unaided.

In the main it was decided therefore, with the approval of our senior staff, to send the prospective researchers, after completion of their clinical residency, to distinguished scientists and basic science departments either at Columbia or elsewhere to continue their training. For example, after doing their initial research in the basic science departments at Columbia both Richard Kitz and S.H. Ngai did a year of graduate study in Stockholm at the Karolinska Institute. Allen Hyman, on the completion of his initial experience in New York, worked with Geoffrey Dawes at Oxford in England. Some of our people worked in a clinical department most commonly the Department of Medicine at Columbia which had more than its fair share of excellent scientists in different fields of study. Among the able people we sent to work in the unit directed by the distinguished scientists Andre Cournand and Dickinson Richards in cardio-pulmonary medicine were Bob Epstein and Stuart Sullivan. Cournand and Richards subsequently won the Nobel Prize for Physiology or Medicine for their work in cardiac catheterization. Lenny Brand spent a year in Copenhagen.

The drawback of the plan was that the scientific portion was sometomes not long enough for major career purposes. Some of the staff had the opportunity to continue their scientific educational experience by working part-time with their mentors after becoming members of our faculty. Richard Kitz had this sort of relationship with Ernie Wilson in biochemistry and S.H. Ngai had it with S.C. Wang in pharmacology. In short we did the best that we could in the same spirit that our clinical decentralization was designed to sharpen and develop expertise among our clinical anesthesiologists by having them maintain relationships with a specific group of experts. It was a broad application of the principle of intellectual and personal contiguity with very able scientists.

There remained the question of the organizational function in research. Should we have a Director of Research? I thought we should.

To implement this decision I invited Dr. Francis F. Foldes to join me from the Mercy Hospital in Pittsburgh where he directed the department of anesthesiology. Dr. Foldes' major career in research in anesthesiologywas recognized later by many highly deserved honors including the Distinguished Award for Research of the American Society of Anesthesiologists. Unfortunately for me (and for the testing of my hypothesis) Dr. Foldes elected not to accept my invitation.

It did not take long before the Columbia Department was recognized in the United States and in Europe as one of the "towers of strength" in academic anesthesiology. The Chairman and members of the faculty served in appropriate ways in the various community, and professional support systems of the specialty, including service on the American Board of Anesthesiology's directorate, the Editorial Boards of Journals, Study Sections in the National Institutes of Health, membership on the National Heart Council of the N.I.H, advisory services for the Food and Drug Administration and several Foundations and participated in policy planning and execution of large research programs for the national interest. The Department therefore was locally effective in clinical care, education, and scientific research, and it was a responsible citizen in the academic anesthesia community for the Nation, and of the Western World.

Naturally, there were problems as well as triumphs. Columbia University was unfortunately one of the notable victims of the Vietnam War. The students revolt on the Morningside Heights Campus, very nearly brought a great educational institution to its knees. These disruptive forces in higher education were of course not unique to Columbia, but Columbia was a major sufferer, and its Anesthesiology Department was no exception.

It was toward the end of this disturbing period that I elected to depart most reluctantly from New York to Miami for other opportunities in the medical academic world. Dr. S.H. Ngai assumed the responsibilities of this Department in a most difficult period. He did almost miraculous work in anticipating the directions of change that would have to be met, and prepared the Department for its next phase. With the arrival of Dr. Henrik Bendixen as Chairman, a new phase in the development of the Columbia Department began.

All of these developments undoubtedly contributed to an interesting attitude on the part of our young people. They carried out delightful, vigorous and vociferous celebrations of the establishment of our departmental independence from surgery in January of 1952. They put on an elaborate show consisting of lyrics written by some of our people and wonderful popular music by the great composers of that era. They were very clever indeed. These performances became annual. They were important occasions. Symbolically, to emphasize the notion of independence, the show was originally performed on Washington's birthday. These annual shows were put on or near Washington's birthday to again symbolize the freedom of independence and to celebrate with great gusto.

These were absolutely marvelous occasions where the spirits ran high and sometimes excessively so! The lyrics, so very cleverly crafted by many of our people were sly and yet wonderful lampoons of the eccentrics in the department and of the peculiar aspects of my leadership, as they saw it, as well as some of the sentimental journeys we took together. These were wonderful occasions and they, among other things, produced a great deal of theatrical originality in addition to very good fellowship amongst us.

Many people contributed to writing the lyrics but outstanding among them certainly were Sol Shnider and Leonard Brand. The department emotionally, intellectually and professionally was now a real extended family.

From the discussion in this chapter it is clear that most of the aspirations for the development and evolution of the Department of Anesthesiology at the Columbia-Presbyterian Medical Center went well. Patient care was always a priority of this department fom the beginning when it was a division of the department of surgery. It continued to evolve and became one of world class excellence and recognized as such by the anesthesiology community. Its research has been only partially described but the method of developing research competence and its collorary, leadership, have been described in detail. One of the department's outstanding accomplishments in the world of its specialty was the development of extraordinarily competent leaders in the field including departmental chairmen, very able clinicians and outstanding scientists.

The Department participated in the teaching program of medical students and of the mutual teaching activities which a distinguished and influential faculty in basic science and clinical medicine exercised with each other. For example the very important Combined Clinic that was organized and managed on a weekly basis by a very strong Department of Medicine included me and other members of our department as presenters of important developments in anesthesiology, clinical pharmacology or other matters that would be of interest to a interdisciplinary faculty. For instance, one of our Combined Clinic presentations included as guests such distinguished scientists as Dr. Bernard Brodie and John Burns. They and other basic science specialists who worked with us, presented with us an analysis of the methods of drug disposition and the methods of drug action in various organs and tissues of the body. These exercises were very well received by the College of Physicians and Surgeons faculty and students.

We felt also that it was our responsibility and opportunity to bring together bright, young and promising scientifically oriented anesthesiologists in appropriate intellectual settings dealing with the science that could be applied to clinical care or had the potential of doing so. We were able to establish the first important international meeting on muscle relaxants which brought together our own Columbia people and experts in the science and clinical application of this work from all parts of the Unites States and abroad — especially the United Kingdom.

A meeting was also held in collaboration with the New York Academy of Medicine that dealt with pharmacokinetics, then known as uptake and distribution of drugs. Many young investigators such as Dr. Edmond Eger II, Dr. Lawrence Saidman and Dr. C. Philip Larson, young people of great promise or actual performance were brought together to discuss with each other and with the young and intellectually bright members of the Columbia department their research work and their attitudes towards its development for the future. A classic book was put together by Dr. Kitz and me on the results of this conference. The book has served as a basis for the subsequent very rapid and impressive development of the science of pharmacokinetics in anesthesiology. An important side effect of this meeting was the subsequent interest of the New York Academy of Medicine in the field of anesthesiology. We were able to persuade this distinguished organization to establish a section devoted to our work. The section of Anesthesiology and Resuscitation, as it was called, was established in the Academy. A further development in spreading the contact relationships of intellectually oriented anesthesiologists with other medical scientists came when anesthesiologists were admitted to fellowship in the American College of Physicians (rather than the American College of Surgeons) as a clear indication that the leaders in Anesthesiology viewed themselves as part of Medicine rather than specialists in Surgery. This was an important development in defining what anesthesiology was and who its people were.

During this period of the expansion of interests in organizational behavior and activities, the Association of University Anesthesiologists was formed. I was one of its original four founders. Most university anesthesiologists are familiar with its history or can easily become so by reading the various articles including my own on its creation. In the course of these evolutionary expansion activities, several members of the department became examiners for the American Board of Anesthesiology for its oral examination and also wrote examination questions for the written examination. I was elected to membership of the Board of Directors of the American Board of Anesthesiology and completed my service as its president.

Many of my Columbia colleagues also served on various committees in the American Society of Anesthesiologists especially those geared towards education and the application of science to clinical care. I participated as well and was elected the president of that society and served in 1968 as its Chief Executive Officer. This work was recognized far and wide by the achievement of important prizes and distinctions by my colleagues. Many of them served in distinguished European and British institutions, e.g. Oxford University, the Karolinska Institute in Stockholm, the University of Uppsala in Sweden, many American institutions and other distinguished academic organizations in the European low countries and on the continent. N.I.H. fellowships were frequently achieved as were fellowships awarded by foundations. Two of my colleagues became Guggenheim Fellows. One of my colleagues, Allen Hyman subsequently became a Robert Wood Johnson Fellow and served in Washington for a year.

I received more than my fair share of honors and recognition including the election to honorary membership in many foreign societies of anesthesiologists. I was also awarded honorary fellowships in the Royal College of Anaesthestists of the United Kingdom, the Faculty of Anaesthesia of the College of Surgeons in Ireland and Honorary Fellowship in the Royal Society of Medicine of England.

In addition to membership and honorary fellowship in many anesthesia societies, I was also awarded honorary doctoral degrees in medicine by the universities of Turin in Italy, Uppsala in Sweden and Vienna in Austria. Columbia University was kind enough to award me an honorary Doctor of Science degree in 1988 which is considerably cherished because of its origins in the institution where I spent so much of my active life and career. Columbia also was generous enough to establish an endowed chair in anesthesiology named for me as a result of their feeling about the work that I had contributed to our department. I view it as evidence of confidence in the history and the development of that department by all my able colleagues rather than my own achievements. This chair was established in 1984 and its first occupant was the distinguished anesthesiologist, Dr. Henrick Bendixen.

At this period I also had the very great pleasure and honor of being a member of the Lasker jury on scientific awards for distinction in basic science and clinical medicine. These awards were highly respected and greatly coveted by scientists and clinicians because they were so exceptionally selective. Many later won the Nobel Prize. I learned very much by being a member of this distinguished jury and served with them for a period of some twenty five years.

SOME PATIENTS I HAVE MET

In the immediate post World War II period and extending for quite a long time toward the end of the twentieth century, the Columbia-Presbyterian Medical Center was very much in its Camelot years. The professional staff both clinical and basic science consisted of outstanding individuals who were highly regarded and respected. The neighborhood in Washington Heights where the Medical Center is placed was a quiet pleasant middle class neighborhood settled in fairly substantial numbers by German-Jewish refugees from Hitler's Europe. Local businesses flourished. It was absolutely safe to walk on the streets at any time day or night. In this environment Dr. Dana Atchley, who had the attributes of a fine scientist, a splendid clinician, a wise philosopher and a most tolerant and open minded leader, attracted many patients to the Medical Center, as did so many of his other colleagues. For all these reasons the Columbia-Presbyterian Medical Center was a Mecca where the wealthy and distinguished people from many parts of the country and the world sought their medical care. Always there was the possibility of divergent attitudes about therapy in which case the patient's physician chose among the richness of advice that he received.

Very early after my arrival my good friend and a most distinguished physician, Dr. Alvan Barach, the man who designed the oxygen tent for the treatment of pneumonia, brought to us a most fascinating patient. However a word or two about Dr. Barach is necessary because it helps explain the course of events that followed. At his peak, in addition to being an expert general internist he was also gifted in the fabrication of instruments and machines that were related to oxygen therapy. He was a great scholar in many areas and also was a highly competent psychoanalyst. In fact he practiced psychoanalysis one day a week as part of his medical care of patients. He was analyzed by the distinguished Franz Alexander in Chicago and remained a close friend of Alexander until the latter's death. I had the privilege of meeting Dr. Alexander through Al Barach and enjoyed the discussion that I was able to witness. Barach also wrote at least one novel under the pseudonym of John Coignard.

This very unusual physician and I became good friends. He felt that excellent anesthesia was a necessity for his patients and he frequently sought me out with the idea that either I would take care of his patient or select the right person if it was an area in which I had not as much competence or experience as one of my colleagues. Early in 1950, Dr. Barach called me and wanted to talk about a patient about whom he was concerned. He wanted me to give the patient anesthesia for an exploratory laporatomy looking for the possibility of a malignant tumor in the colon. In those days, I must hasten to add, resources such as colonoscopy were not yet available. Laporatomy, it had to be. So, many patients had to undergo exploration which happily today is not necessary any longer. That was the surgical problem. Next was the problem related to anesthesia. The patient we were concerned about was Mr. Charles B. Wrightsman. He was the wonderful individual who became a very dear friend and also was the supporter financially and conceptually of my trip to various institutions to see what good anesthesiology programs were like and strengthen our own at the Columbia-Presbyterian Medical Center.

Mr. Wrightsman was deeply concerned about anesthesia. This problem was not unique in 1950 because of the way in which anesthesia had been administered to a fair number of people when they were small and defenseless children. Charles Wrightsman had the experience, as a very young child, of being held forcefully against his will on a table in the kitchen of his home so that he could be etherized for the removal of his tonsils. He remembered vividly the deep feeling of anxiety and helplessness that he experienced as a young child in being so forcefully restrained and being smothered, by an unknown stranger. He was not old enough to know that it was allegedly for his own good! He carried this unfortunate fear most his life. Actually the problem he presented to Dr. Barach and to me was not a rare one but it was rare to find somebody with such intelligence being able to describe it as vividly as he did. Dr. Barach knew perfectly well that this issue had to be solved before we could deal with the basic problem of diagnosis and appropriate therapy for the polyp he had in his colon. Al Barach was very astute and recognized that this problem resulted in Mr. Wrightsman's signing himself out of several hospitals because he was unable to face being anesthetized, in the way he expected it would be. He thought it would be a reprise of his childhood experience. He was of course unaware that the anesthesia advances by 1950 could avoid all unpleasantness for him and that he would not have to experience the anxiety of being smothered.

After being thoroughly alerted to the nature of the problem I went to see our patient and listened to an extraordinary story of his childhood experiences. After absorbing all the details, I assured him that he would be unaware of any discomfort with respect to the administration of anesthesia and in fact would not even recall being anesthetized.

Mr. Wrightsman had no trouble with the use of needles so that it was comfortable and easy for him to have an intravenous drip started and secured in place in his room. Small doses of thiopental were administered until he lost consciousness. He was then transported to the operating room where a benign polyp was removed from his colon.

There were no recovery rooms at the time at the Medical Center and he was taken straight away to his room where I stayed with him until he became conscious. When he awoke he was unaware of anything having occurred and asked when we would be doing the operation. The success of our effort was obviously a great happiness to him when he was far enough along in the recovery after surgical treatment to realize that he had escaped all of the unpleasantness about which he was concerned. As I write this short description of what was described as "stealing" an operation for a patient's comfort I am amazed at how simple procedures can produce profound effects. This is but one small example of the major advances that have occurred for the benefit of patients in the administration of anesthesia. During the recovery period, which took place in his room, he was very comfortable and delighted to know that he did not have a malignant tumor and that all was well.

Much to my delight, this was the beginning of a very happy and wonderful friendship for me and I think a good and useful one for him as well. He was much interested in what he termed the magic of modern anesthesia and wanted to help develop it.

Charles Wrightsman supported me with his friendship and also also expressed it by financial support of my own research and that of my colleagues. In short, he got us off to a very good start, so that we could compete successfully in the national arena for grant support for research. His interest in my activities continued until his death. There is no way in which I can ever show my gratitude sufficiently for the many things that he did for my professional and personal welfare.

Charlie invited me every winter to take a week or so of rest and recreation at his beautiful home in Palm Beach, Florida during the winter. Every February I spent some time at the beautiful Wrightsman home where the food was magnificent, the courtesy and friendship of Charlie and his wonderful wife Jayne were marvelous for me to experience.

The Wrightsmans often had guests of prominence in the business or the professional worlds and in the world of the arts, to which they were both very much devoted. I saw beautiful people and beautiful things at their home and learned a great deal about a realm that was new to me and most attractive. I had such lovely experiences as playing tennis with Mr. Allen Dulles; talking at length with the distinguished director of the Metropolitan Museum of Art, Philippe de Montebello; many trustees of the Metropolitan Museum who were also distinguished leaders in New York's society and an occasional political figure of importance like the future President of the United States, John F. Kennedy. All of these fantastic experiences contributed in a major way to my growth and development in that I could see with considerable clarity how life in the world of art, business and professional activities fitted together. One aspect could nourish and support the other. One did not have to be a physician with narrow tubular vision in order to enjoy one's professional work but could enjoy as well the worlds of the arts, literature, and business.

Often during the summers Charles and Jayne invited me to spend two weeks visiting various places in the Mediterranean which could be comfortably reached by a beautiful and glorious yacht called Radiant II. Each summer we went to a different part of the Mediterranean and we were always prepared for the sights that were to be seen by doing "homework" arranged by Charles and provided in written form for each of his guests. The guides to the various places that we visited were usually scholars with great knowledge about the areas that we toured. In the course of several such visits I saw many of the glories of classical Greece, of Asia Minor, North Africa and the southern parts of Italy., and many wonderful things along the Adriatic near the coast of the former Yugoslavia. It was a superlative and breathtaking experience to sail on so luxurious a yacht with modest numbers of extraordinarily interesting people.

During our visits we stopped to dine with some of the most attractive people who were friends of the Wrightsmans. In one such visit we dined with Lord and Lady Rothschild and the Duke of Marlborough. Lord Rothschild was one of the world's experts on avian reproduction, especially the biology of avian spermatozoa. I learned a great deal about an aspect of biology of which I never knew anything at all before. The Duke of Marlborough bore a strong resemblance to Winston Churchill. The present Duke of Marlborough is a direct descendant of General John Churchill who was created a Duke by Queen Anne to celebrate a great British victory over Louis XIV at Blenheim. Sir Winston Churchill was a member of this family and in fact was born at the ancestral home of the Dukes of Marlborough.

Another very good friendship also came to me from a patient whom I had met at the Columbia-Presbyterian Medical Center. This was the distinguished founder of the advertising and public relations business, Mr. Albert D. Lasker. Unfortunately Mr. Lasker's death occurred soon after our friendship began. However, I had the singular good fortune of having the friendship of his widow, the very able and important contributor to medical research support and welfare in the United States, Mary W. Lasker. Much more will be said about her in connection with my experience with the National Institutes of Health in Washington. A part of the story of looking after Mr. Lasker and administering anesthesia to him concerns the medical care of Very Important Persons.

Albert Lasker was a member of a prominent family from Galveston, Texas. He was scheduled for operation by Dr. Fordyce B. St. John (the same distinguished surgeon who operated on Charles Wrightsman) for a tumor of the colon. Mr. Lasker had a misfortune which he shared with several of his siblings. They had the same disease and died of cancer of the colon. His operation resulted in palliative care but not in the cure of the malignant tumor. However this tale is not similar to that of Mr. Wrightsman. It is more a reflection on some sociological aspects of the surgical treatment of very distinguished and powerful patients.

Mr. Lasker was seen and treated by many consultants in the course of his illnesses. His importance was expressed in a most interesting and fairly extravagant way on the day he was scheduled for his operation. Mr. Lasker was brought up to the operating room and put in an anesthesia induction room (we had them at that time and it was one of our largest ones). In addition to the surgical team consisting of Dr. St. John, the senior surgeon and his long time friend, colleague and always first assistant, Dr.

Rudolph Schullinger, there were two other assistants who were residents. Present, also were many of the Chairmen of the various Columbia departments including those of Medicine, Urology and several others. The anesthesia induction room was completely packed by a solicitous group of very distinguished physicians and their assistants. Present was Dr. Robert F. Loeb (Chairman of our Department of Medicine) and George Cahill (our important and influential Chairman of the Department of Urology) and, of course, Mr. Lasker's personal physician, the vital and distinguished Dr. Dana Atchley. All of these people so crowded the anesthesia induction room that there was no room for me to do anything to begin anesthesia. Also, as Albert Lasker was comfortably conversing with several of them, it seemed rude of me to interrupt them .

So I went outside the induction room and sat down on a stool just trying to think of what to do next. While all this was taking place, Dr. St. John came around and found me and asked whether there was any reason that I wasn't starting. His concern, quite properly, was that perhaps I had found something about Mr. Lasker that we needed to attend to before beginning anesthesia. Dr. St. John was always very courteous, very kind and very friendly and his inquiry was in that spirit. I told him of my problem that there were so many people in the induction room that it was not only impossible for me to get near Mr. Lasker to start but that it was probably unsafe for so many people in various stages of inappropriate garb to be in that part of our operating room area. He laughed and certainly eased my concern. The next thing I knew is that there was a long line of very important colleagues and distinguished physicians and surgeons streaming out of the induction room to the observing gallery which was on the floor above us. All this consumed almost a half hour until things were sorted out correctly. I then began anesthesia and there were no further complications either sociological or medical to describe.

I could not help but speculate later on the meaning of the traffic jam that I encountered in the induction room. I can suggest two important possibilities. The first, the one that I think was the explanation, is that many people were consulted in Albert Lasker's care and they were all attracted by this exceptionally bright and engaging person. They wanted to do all they could to help him in sustaining him in what must have been a difficult experience. The other possibility is that each of the experts and consultants had to "earn his keep" and demonstrate his closeness to the patient by appearing in the scene where none of them was needed. Some "unfair" people might consider the second a more appropriate explanation for what happened but I rather think not. It is amusing however to speculate on the dynamics of patient care when the patient is a real V.I.P.

One Saturday, I was summoned from a meeting of the Post Graduate Assembly in Anesthesiology in downtown Manhattan to return to the Medical Center to provide anesthesia for Elizabeth Taylor, the famous actress of the cinema world. She had a herniated disc and Dr. Lester Mount was going to operate on her that weekend because the viability of the large sciatic nerve was threatened by pressure from the disc. The operation and anesthesia were relatively uneventful but the post operative care had a major effect upon me. Ms. Taylor's then husband, Michael Todd, had her room filled with wonderful impressionist paintings of very great value. Also, I was smitten by her incredibly beautiful violet colored eyes. I was considerably surprised to note that there was some small evidence of what I interpreted as vitiligo on some of the skin of her face. If that diagnosis was correct, the make-up people had done a superb job for her film photography. She was incredibly beautiful and very nice and pleasant to talk with. The final aspect of caring for her was when she was discharged from the hospital somehow her husband "forgot" the valuable paintings and they had to be retrieved.

Ambassador Averill Harriman was also a patient. He was a former Governor of New York and an occasional would-be candidate for the Democratic nomination for the presidency of the United States. Ambassador Harriman was a very tall distinguished looking man and always made extremely good sense.

He was very cordial, very correct, and very friendly in all our dealings. By that time however he had grown quite deaf and it was not easy to talk with him. Harriman was also a patient of Dr. Barach's and all went exceedingly well with his anesthesia and operation.

A patient with whom I had some technical problems was the wonderful singer, Edith Piaf, who came to Dr. George Humphreys as a patient from Paris. She was thin, almost scrawny and yet wonderful in her demeanor. What I did not know but what probably many other people knew was that she was a "main line shooter" of drugs and the result was a severe scarring of almost all her peripheral veins of both upper extremities, which I needed for intravenous fluids as well as for the induction of anesthesia.

Mme. Piaf saw my difficulty right away and volunteered to insert the needle for me into one her veins which she knew was accessible. I therefore became one of the very few people I know about who was assistant anesthesiologist for induction purposes to a distinguished singer and actress! She was so skillful at intravenous placement of needles that I had no further difficulty with her.

Another patient of extraordinary interest was that great lady Mrs. Eleanor Roosevelt, the widow of President Franklin D. Roosevelt. Mrs. Roosevelt presented a problem that I never met before I looked after her, nor afterward. She had to have an operation upon her hand and wanted to have no drugs that would interfere with her sensorium or in any way inhibit her working with her secretary after the operation was over. Her surgeon, Dr. McLaughlin, told me from what he knew of her that that was entirely feasible for her to do — so strong was her disciplined self will. In accordance with her wishes I therefore elected to use no pre-anesthetic medication and gave her a brachial plexus block. She required no medication during the operation and upon its completion once again refused to have any medication for pain, discomfort or for sedation. She asked also not to be sent to the recovery room and went back to her own room where her secretary was waiting for her. As soon as Mrs. Roosevelt was settled in bed she began to work with her secretary. Her post operative course was totally uneventful and the experience had an indelible effect upon my mind. I had never seen so delightful, strong and interesting a patient who pretty much directed the traffic her way and had it work very well.

Cole Porter was a patient who required repeated operations for osteomyelitis. It was difficult to deal with Mr. Porter because he was in discomfort bordering on severe chronic pain. The delightful spirit I expected of the composer of so many wonderful songs and bright lyrics was unhappy in the hospital. The professional output of the individual may not necessarily reflect a true persona or vice versa depending on the influence of disease, pain, injury or illness on personality. I never knew, therefore, what the true Cole Porter was like. My sympathies went to him although it was always difficult to try to take care of his needs We were not very effective in controlling his pain between operations.

Another patient who had a great impact upon me and my growth and development was Madame Chiang-Kai-Chek whose story was a very different one for us. Her medical care was often performed at the Columbia-Presbyterian Medical Center but this particular episode required our traveling to Taiwan because Madame did not feel she could leave Taiwan even to get her gall bladder removed, which was necessary in the light of her surgical diagnosis and prognosis.

Her surgeon was our professor of surgery, Dr. George Humphreys and he asked me to accompany him to give anesthesia to Madame Chiang in Taipei, which I agreed to do with some misgiving. The misgiving was based upon the fact that I had always been cautioned by my good friends who taught and worked internationally, as I had begun to do, to try to avoid operating in a strange environment unless you could control all the factors, such as operating room personnel, the nature of instruments and the provision of the right kind of anesthetic apparatus and supplies. Although everything was possible in the Taiwan of the Generalissimo's regime it still was not a certainty.

George Humphreys was quite sure we could do all right and although he had somewhat similar feelings about equipment and people he had much more experience with China and its people than I did. He said that he would be very happy if I went with him to Taiwan. I decided to go. We checked out all the things we could about apparatus, instruments and the like before we went and were assured that everything would be in great shape. That was mistake number one. A second consideration was what would happen if things went wrong for any reason. Being in a dictator's small country was not a comfortable experience and this possibility, although it never amounted to anything serious, was potential mistake number two.

On arrival at Taipei after a very pleasant although long airplane trip, George and I were happily ensconced in a beautiful little house where we had our own servants and chef. We were summoned by Mme. Chiang almost immediately for tea.

I was struck with how very beautiful this lady was in what I thought to be old age (I have since learned that my judgment is grossly incorrect about the age of anybody especially of beautiful, intelligent and brilliant women). She was very glad to see us; greeted us warmly over tea and again to my surprise spoke beautiful American Southern English which I certainly did not expect despite our preparations ahead of time. Mme. Chiang went to Wellesley College after living many of her speech-forming years in the American South. Beauty, brains and charm ruled her universe as far as I was concerned and I think George Humphreys agreed. However we were beginning to become restive after a couple of days in that no time could be set for the operation for reasons totally unknown to us. We pressed the point since Mme. Chiang had brought us all this distance to operate upon her. We wanted a firm date for the operation or else there wasn't much point in our simply being treated to a vacation of sorts even though it was a pleasant and enjoyable time. She apparently gave way as to setting a date. It was only later that we found out that France had recognized the People's Republic of China and this was a bad sign for Mme. Chiang in that it suggested there would be a whole host of undesirable political changes. Eventually, the People's Republic of China would become recognized and the regime of Chiang and his people of the Republic of China would be ousted from the Security Council of the United Nations. This was, an important political event and it was one of the reasons why the operation was delayed for a few days. When she agreed a very unusual thing occurred and never before nor since has it happened in my experience.

It was decided to operate upon her in the Veteran's Administration Hospital's which was a very lovely place. In some ways it resembled our Veteran's Administration Hospital but in others it was quite different. There was a very comfortable almost palatial suite of rooms that was dedicated obviously to very important personages. But what was unusual in my experience was that the entire hospital seemed to have been emptied when Mme. Chiang was to be operated upon, possibly as a security precaution for her welfare against a possible assassination as well as for her husband's. It didn't occur to me until later but it was possible that both George Humphreys and I could have been in a precarious situation if things went wrong. It was better to have an empty hospital for us as well as for them for similar security purposes.

Before leaving New York I had conferred with my very close friend and splendid colleague, Dr. S.H. Ngai about Taiwan. My reason for discussing things with Dr. Ngai was that his father-in-law had been an official in Generalissimo Chiang's cabinet and might know something of value to me. The political events were not too important to us as it turned out, but Dr. Ngai cautioned me about the importance of recognizing anesthetic problems in people of Chinese ancestry. They seemed to be, for reasons not at that time determined, more susceptible to analgesic and to anesthetic drugs than were Caucasian people. I must say that I took his advice seriously because of his brilliance but I really did not expect to see how accurate he was in terms of the effect of opiate analgesics upon Mme. Chiang when we actually did the operation. We didn't have any problems with anesthesia or surgery which went well including the happy assistance provided to us by surgical and anesthetic physicians during the cholecystectomy.

It was a relatively new idea at the time that it was possible to provide good post operative analgesia with a continuous epidural block. I attempted to achieve this with equipment that was inadequate for the purpose (error number three). I produced a flow of spinal fluid, a "wet tap." I therefore thought it was unsafe to provide epidural analgesia for Mme. Chiang and did not try to do it. Much to my delight, however she had very little pain post operatively and I would have erroneously attributed her comfort to the block had it been used. She was an extraordinary woman, determined to get back into the controlling areas that she exercised in the political life of Taiwan. She would brook no interference from post operative recovery or from post operative pain.

George Humphreys and I received suitable gifts from Mme. Chiang for our care and probably the most precious one to me was the opportunity to see the great treasures that Generalissimo Chiang had taken from mainland China to Taiwan when the Communists secured control of the mainland. These treasures at the time were kept in caves for security as well as for artistic conservation purposes. All this occurred before the beautiful museum was built in Taipei to house these treasures.

In addition to caring for Mme. Chiang we had the great pleasure of seeing Sidney and Elaine Blumenthal, Columbia's distinguished pediatric cardiologist and his wife. They were doing a sabbatical leave's work in Taipei. He was a very good friend of ours. Pediatric cardiology was always very important to George since he was much occupied with and interested in the surgical treatment of children with cardio-vascular disease. Our return to New York was most pleasant. George and I became very close friends.

Another patient who provided me with the kind of experience not to be encountered in any place other than an institution like the Columbia-Presbyterian Medical Center was the Duchess of Windsor.

Her Grace, the Duchess of Windsor, was born an American, Wallis Warfield Simpson. She was, as is well known, twice divorced and therefore unacceptable to the British Royal Family as a spouse for the man who became King Edward VIII. The romance between the then Mrs. Simpson and the then Prince of Wales had no interesting medical aspects but of course it excited the romantic fantasies of the entire world. It ultimately resulted in the abdication of the King who chose to leave his throne so that he could "marry the woman I love." During the War period the former King who assumed the title of Duke of Windsor served in a relatively minor capacity as Governor-General of one of Britain's Caribbean possessions. After the war the Duke and the Duchess moved to Paris where they lived except for the travels to which they had become accustomed including rather frequent visits to their friends in Palm Beach, Florida. They were not permitted to return to the British Isles by the Duke's successor who was his younger brother, who had assumed the title of George VI on his accession to the Throne. To a world interested in these kinds of love affairs the Duke and Duchess were precious people. They were frequent guests and much honored by the international society to which they belonged.

When the Duchess required gynecological attention, she was cared for and treated by Dr. Benjamin Watson who had recently retired from the position of Chairman of the Department of Obstetrics and Gynecology, as was the custom in those days on attaining the age of sixty five. Dr. Watson however, was a doughty Scot who continued his very large and interesting private practice, a custom which was also approved in the 1940s and the 1950s. Private practice permission required concurrence of the current Chairman of the Department and it was renewable year by year until the age of sixty eight when it required the concurrence of the Board of Trustees in addition to the approval of the Chairman. These measures were put into place to be sure that practicing physicians and surgeons were professionally competent and would pose no risk to their patients as they aged. Dr. Watson was more than professionally competent. He was outstanding and an exceptionally gifted gynecological surgeon.

His assistant called me one day to ask whether I could give anesthesia to a patient of importance to Dr. Watson. The patient was in good health except that she required a hysterectomy for her gynecological ailment. He asked me not to divulge the nature of the ailment and I have not done so to this day. Accordingly, the scheduling process was arranged, also at Dr. Watson's request, to be on a day when normal elective surgery was not being done since he wanted his patient to have the kind of security and privacy that he felt was necessary since she was a most glamorous woman who had received much press and other world wide attention at frequent intervals.

I suggested to him that we should pick Washington's birthday which was then celebrated singly rather than as part of a President's birthday holiday combining Washington's and Lincoln's natal days. So February 22nd it was and it was a very happy occasion for me and my colleagues in the Department of Anesthesiology. You will recall that we celebrated our "independence" from the Department of Surgery as symbolic of the spirit of independence on Washington's birthday. I was therefore free to work and concentrate entirely on Dr. Watson and his patient's requirements before going to our annual celebration which took place in the evening. Since there were no other operations, except emergency procedures, on our dockets for that day I also had the not very common but most welcome pleasure of having one of my senior colleagues, Dr. William Howland, assist me in providing anesthesia for the Duchess of Windsor.

The preoperative preparations had an interest that can only be described as social rather than medical or surgical. The Duchess was admitted to a very pleasant and relatively large room in Harkness Pavilion which was where our private patients were housed before, during and after their illnesses or surgical treatment. She had her own dishes and silverware and she very carefully supervised the food that she ate even though it was easily compatible with the medical requirements of an appropriate diet prior to an operation such as hysterectomy. This is the lady who is widely quoted as saying: "You can never be too rich nor too thin." To accompany the interesting diet and the plates and silverware were her very beautiful and lovely bed sheets, night apparel and similar objects familiar to her. She always had a maid in attendance who was very competent and also very pleasant. There were no difficulties in performing all the required medical, pre-anesthetic and pre-surgical preparations.

On Washington's birthday, the Duchess was brought to the operating room. I anesthetized her with general anesthesia (the anesthetic agents long since forgotten and the chart not easy to obtain if possible at all) she did well and the surgery proceeded along without any undue incident. The end of the story is an interesting touch of wit by Dr. Watson. As he was delivering the Duchess' uterus into the wound for removal he looked at me, looked at the specimen, looked at all his assistants and the nurses and he said "I want all of you to remember that this is what very nearly disturbed beyond repair the entire British Empire." The Duchess went on to an uneventful recovery from the surgery. I had the pleasure of meeting her one subsequent time with her husband at a mutual friend's home in Palm Beach. Her memory of Dr. Watson and me was, to say the least, somewhat vague. However she was very pleasant and acknowledged that it had been an easy experience for her.

Most of my clinical experiences were neither with famous nor exciting people. They were important to me, but not necessarily to the rest of the world. I spent a great deal of time working with surgical residents on their patients who were ward patients. In some institutions they were called "charity" patients. Both these designations are somewhat patronizing and do not really convey the fact that we were delighted to take care of them but there were some caveats. The surgical resident who controlled the ward and the operating schedule for these patients, generally speaking, was more persuaded to admit them when they were patients with "interesting" problems. This practice meant different things for different surgical residents. Usually it meant that the patients needed a complicated surgical procedure or had a difficult problem which required solution. Also, quite often, the patients were very sick and required special and intensive types of surgical treatment.

New surgical procedures were always being performed at this great medical center. Often, morbidity and mortality were high at first and had to be brought to acceptable levels with knowledge and experience. I frequently worked with our surgeons, especially in the early years, to improve our results with better anesthesia care. I also taught younger people what I learned. These patients were often very sick. They were usually poor. They presented ethical dilemmas of various sorts to us in that it was a difficult thing to know when we had gathered enough knowledge from other people's experiences, from research or from laboratory tests to justify performing a new or rarely used surgical procedures on our patients. Often the justification was a fairly obvious one. If something new and different was not available, these patients might die in a short time. Another was the fact that their quality of life could be vastly improved if the operations were successful.

Cardiac surgery is a case in point. It is now commonly performed in most community hospitals even though there is some argument in professional circles about the ethical justification of doing so. The point I wish to make is that it is commonplace enough because many surgeons are qualified and educated properly to do them. Many anesthesiologists have had the requisite experience and it is accepted as an non-experimental process in today's surgical world. However it was not always thus.

We began our open heart surgery program in the early phases of knowledge in that particular field. We felt unjustified in offering these procedures to any but the most desperately ill patients who, of course, added much morbidity and mortality to our outcomes. We did the best we could. All the procedures and their risks were explained to the patients in very great detail.

Not everybody was willing to accept the risks despite the fact that no other therapies could be considered useful. The surgeon in charge of this program was my closest friend for a good many years, Dr. Aaron Himmelstein. He got the program off to as good a start as one could expect with all the uncertainties of the time. Our mortality record was not good at the outset. Our experience was a humbling one to me and to him. There was even a time when I felt that we should stop the program and wait for more research information. Aaron did not agree, and the results started to improve enough to encourage us.

As the program began to shape up a tragedy occurred. Aaron Himmelstein became ill with a brain tumor which killed him in a relatively short time. It was a great loss for me — my best friend and my closest professional colleague — at the time we were working to put a cardiac surgery program on its feet. Aaron's successor, Dr. James Malm was just completing his residency but was a very gifted young surgeon who continued Aaron's wonderful work and made the Columbia-Presbyterian Medical Center an outstanding one for cardiac surgery. By then, Stuart Sullivan and Dick Patterson were competent at cardiac anesthesia. They soon replaced me in the program.

Early in my experience at the Medical Center we were doing large blood vessel surgery such as correction of aortic aneurysm and here too our patients were far from famous and far from well to do. We evolved a program that became very respectable in a relatively short time and learned much that we were able to transmit to our colleagues in surgery and anesthesiology. Arthur Voorhees led our surgical group and Richard Kitz our anesthesiology group in performing these procedures. The results were published and were helpful to others.

Our muscle relaxant program aided many aspects of surgical therapy. Ron Katz, Aaron Gissen and Hans Karis were responsible for the achievements. Raymond Fink added greatly to our knowledge of the larynx in his pioneering and brilliant study of the structure and functions of that organ. He contributed in an important way to the development of our monitoring capabilities as well. He also designed an excellent non-breathing valve and began his important work on local anesthetic agents. Fink's great creativity matured further when he joined the Department of Anesthesiology at the University of Washington in Seattle under the leadership of the late Dr. John Bonica.

Another area in which many patients came to us because of our superior knowledge was in the field now known as surgery for endocrinological disorders. A most interesting one was operative removal of pheochromocytoma. These tumors were in the adrenal glands or in other chromaffin tissue. They produce epinephrine or norepinephrine which enters the blood stream. The hormones in these tumors could be destructively dangerous. It took very great skill in surgical treatment and in anesthetic management to avoid pushing large amounts of epinephrine into the blood stream and causing serious cardiovascular dysfunction or collapse. We learned how to manage these difficult cases with the Chairman of the Department of Urology, the very able surgeon Dr. George Cahill. Dr. Apgar and I began our anesthetic management of these patients. Soon others of our group participated.

Not all of the patients in our earliest years were famous and distinguished except in their medical ailments. Many had little or no money. The sociological aspects of my clinical work therefore spread over the entire gamut of the human condition in the United States during the slightly over two decades that I spent at this distinguished institution. Obviously the professional experience was magnificent and the sociological spread ranged from patients who were poor, very sick and in need of the benefits of the latest advances in biomedical science to patients who may or may not have been very sick but by various standards applied to the human condition were famous or important or distinguished. It was a fabulous world with every possible opportunity to be useful to patients who needed every clinical and scientific skill for their anesthetic care. It was truly the Camelot years of anesthetic clinical care.

We performed an average of twenty five thousand operations annually. We had a broad spectrum of anesthetic experiences. We cared for patients with all kinds of medical and surgical problems. The patients came from all walks of life, but most of them were solid middle class people. We had many poor people to treat. We also had more than our fair share of the rich and famous. My colleagues and I responded with happy alacrity to our opportunity to support and expand the Camelot years at the Columbia-Presbyterian Medical Center.

A MEDICAL MISSION FOR ANESTHESIOLOGY IN WASHINGTON

One bright day in early 1964 I received an invitation from Dr. H. Houston Merritt, the Dean of the Faculty at Columbia's College of Physicians and Surgeons, i.e. my boss, to see him. Dr. Merritt was a brilliant neurologist and one of the greatest of human beings. All of us highly respected him and also loved him a great deal. He was a distinguished leader and a very good friend to his faculty. I was very proud indeed to have a share in his friendship during the years he was Chief Executive Officer of our School of Medicine.

Houston asked me if I had ever taken a sabbatical leave and I responded that I had not. He suggested that it might be time to have one and I was beginning to get a little bit nervous. I wondered, for example, whether he felt that he needed to have me disappear for six months or a year in view of the various commotions that I might have caused, but I should have known better. He wanted me to go to Washington and serve in the National Institutes of Health as a consultant to Dr. Fred Stone in order to develop certain programs that were considered important. He felt that the time had come where at least one new Institute should be created for the frank support of basic science and its related clinical activities. Another example he gave me was the difficulty in fields such as anesthesiology of attracting the right kind of help and support because of its comparative anonymity to the profession, to scientists as well as to the consuming public. I asked whether I might have a talk with Fred Stone before I agreed to go to Washington and of course Dr. Merritt said that it was entirely possible and that it should be done. But I did not know at the time that Fred had specifically asked for me to serve with him because we had done some things together that pleased him and he thought I could be helpful to him and the N.I.H.. Accordingly I had several very satisfactory and very agreeable long talks with Fred about the fact that Dean Merritt wanted me to spend a sabbatical leave of whatever length of time it took, presumably not to exceed one year, to help in the mission that was of interest to Fred, the establishment of a National Institute of General Medical Sciences. This institute if approved by Congress would subserve the research interests of the basic sciences as well as some of the clinical fields that needed special attention. Fred agreed. My chief interest was, of course, the establishment of research support for anesthesiology.

I recognized, after some discussion with Fred Stone and some of his colleagues that there was also a very important need for the support of research in surgery, radiology, pathology and pharmacology. Fred asked whether I would be willing to serve as his Principal Consultant and spend at least six months, and more if necessary, to establish the new Institute and also to get support via the mechanisms of the National Institutes of Health which would require a good deal of work on many levels. The fact that Jim Shannon was the Director of the National Institutes of Health was a blessing for me since, it may be recalled, I had been a graduate student in Homer Smith's department where part of my work was to assist Jim Shannon in his research at the time he was a senior faculty member in the distinguished and important Department of Physiology at New York University. After the preliminary discussions, I agreed to go to Washington as the Principal Consultant to Fred Stone and to the Institute which would be established in due course. Fred Stone quite understandably took this as a franchise to support not only basic science but any field that seemed to be an orphan and deserved attention for the benefit of the national welfare.

I moved to Bethesda, Maryland in the early part of 1964 in order to spend full time in working with Fred and his colleagues. It turned out to be a fascinating and exhilarating experience but it was very hard work. We knew no boundaries of time and went on from very early in the morning to very late at night on most occasions. Fred Stone was a brilliant N.I.H. executive and administrator and understood very well how to craft his programs. He was of great help to me in producing the ones we had agreed to support. He was also fantastically able in understanding how support systems could be developed that would provoke little or no opposition. We were very successful in getting approval from "Building One," Jim Shannon's office as Director. He was also of enormous help in educating me on how to testify before Congress and its committees and how to put together proposals that were honest and true and would help promote the health of the nation in the most important sense of that word.

The National Institute of General Medical Sciences was recommended through channels by the administration and strongly supported by the President. It was in fairly short order approved by the Congress and the new Institute was established. It turned out to be a matter of great encouragement to basic scientists who had always felt neglected and understandably so. The various institutes that had preceded the National Institute of General Medical Sciences all dealt with a disease or a collection of diseases. Basic scientists felt that they had to subvert their talents for untrammeled research to clinical events. This was now a new and a clear franchise for our most important research organization, the N.I.H., to develop basic sciences regardless of their immediate applicability to patient care problems. Patient Care always remained important to the nation's welfare but it was recognized at long last that tscientific research unlimited except by creativity or lack thereof was now a legitimate and established part of the nation's activities in biomedical science. It also became the home, as I mentioned previously, of those clinical disciplines that seemed to find no natural haven in the disease oriented older institutes.

In addition to working full time with Fred Stone and members of his staff I received very helpful and important advice from Mike Gorman ,who was responsible for the Lasker Foundation interests on a national level and was Mary Lasker's main staff representative in Washington. One of his tasks was to help people who were to testify before Congress — usually distinguished clinicians or scientists — prepare their testimony and become effective witnesses for the public welfare in matters of health and related interests. I received a full course of education from Mike on how to testify to bring the important aspects of what we were advocating to the attention of Congress.

Fred and I, in developing the program for anesthesiology, decided to present its mortality data as a danger to the public health of the nation. The consensus opinion about anesthesia mortality at the end of World War II was that approximately one in six thousand anesthetized patients died because something went wrong due to the anesthesia. Although there was incomplete agreement on what an anesthetic death was, nonetheless the consensus about the rate of mortality was remarkably clear. The difficulty was that not all experts agreed. The experts did not agree on whether anesthetic death was only due to errors or whether there is some intrinsic non-manageable part of the anesthetic interaction with the human body that may cause death. There was disagreement over the role of error and even state of knowledge about a given anesthetic subject. Also the actual denominator of the fraction which reflects the total numbers of anesthetics was unknown. Nobody knew exactly how many anesthetics were given. The reporting of precise numbers was limited to different state jurisdictions and institutions but did not include anesthesia in dentists' offices and other places that aren't counted in hospital reports of anesthetic and surgical procedures. Despite all these difficulties, consensus opinion was as I have described. To me and to many of my colleagues there was an unacceptably high mortality and the way to attack, it we decided, was to improve greatly the education of anesthesiologists in the knowledge that was available and how to use it for patient care. This was a first step that could be initiated institutionally without the necessity of major federal support. However we felt very strongly that the mortality rate due to anesthesia was so unacceptable as to be considered a public health hazard and that really significant progress was dependent upon the acquisition of important new knowledge which means, of course, research.

The program with which I was involved was the securing of adequate support for research in anesthesiology to ameliorate the unacceptable mortality rate of the time. The development of research consisted in the establishment of professional life time workers called career professorships. Another device was the use of career development awards to individuals who had promise and potential of become good scientists in anesthesiology. These awards were usually given for a period of five years and were renewable upon application and performance achievements. Another program that was established in addition to the individual grant support which was the backbone of National Institutes Health's support of research was the creation of program project grants. These dealt with certain fields e.g. anesthesiology research, in which institutions would be awarded grants to support research in certain programmatic areas and also support the people who were engaged in these research activities as well as providing the equipment and other resources for performing research successfully. These program project grants were to be awarded competitively only to institutions who could satisfy all of thee strict requirements. Program project support was crucial in improving anesthetic research and therefore patient care. It was *the* catalyst to making anesthetic care safe and comfortable.

The way these activities and programs were activated was also of interest. After they had been crafted, developed and submitted to review and criticism by leaders in the field they were given back to me and to Fred Stone to formulate new proposals for the National Institutes of Health. We developed a position paper requesting from institutions proposals specifying the approximate number of people who were needed and were qualified to receive the support, the budget arrangements for the program and the method of our providing advice to successful awardees on how to mount and administer their programs. After all these matters were reduced to writing and ready for the approval of the Director, Fred or I brought them to Jim Shannon for his concurrence and suggestions and guidance for necessary revisions. Either Fred or I visited Jim for this function and when we received his approval it was incorporated in the N.I.H. request to the administration for budget support. The process involved our doing appropriate testifying and lobbying to get Congressional approval and passage of these elements of the new recommendations from the N.I.H. Various leaders, including me, were asked to testify before the Congress and were given advice on how to prepare their testimony.

Mary Lasker played a very important part in guiding me and others in how to do the testifying. She arranged for us to dine with members of the appropriate Committees in the Senate or the House of Representatives who were informed that they would get some insight into the new programs coming from N.I.H. under the most pleasant of circumstances. We were delighted to have the opportunity in such favorable environments of explaining and justifying our causes to the senior members and committee chairmen of both houses of Congress. Fellow guests at those Lasker dinner parties often were Senator Lister Hill and Representative John Fogarty, the Chairmen of the key committees in the Senate and in the House of Representatives.

This process continued amicably for all of the initial phases of the support system instituted for the basic sciences and for the five clinical departments (considering pharmacology in its clinical aspects as a clinical department) so that very many important new projects were approved and activated with considerable speed. Fred Stone very generously stated for the public record that our collective work was accomplished in under a year. Normally it could have taken as long as five years to a decade to accomplish, if things had gone along in the usual way with the understandably slow process needed to educate all concerned with the N.I.H. amomg the staff and members of the

Congressional Committees of both Houses. The hastening of the process produced an important program in anesthesiology and very generous funding from the N.I.H. as early as the end of the first budget cycle after the details were all worked out. Large research support was sorely needed and was accorded.

The net result of all of these activities was a very rapid improvement in the knowledge required for a major lowering of the consensus estimate about mortality due to anesthesia. The N.I.H., industry and people who used the newly developed electronic knowledge for monitoring devices all deserved and received adequate credit for the remarkable speed of development of the research which they sponsored. In a relatively short time mortality due to anesthesia was sharply reduced from the one in five or six thousand level to as little as one in four hundred thousand administrations of anesthesia. It was a noteworthy improvement in public health. One expert in public health matters, Dr. George Silver, estimates that, if the consensus aspects are at least reasonably close to the truth, the results of the improvements in anesthesia alone saved the lives of well over one million people anesthetized and operated upon in the United States in the last thirty years.

The research support also had other very important consequences for anesthesiology's development. Bright young people became attracted to the specialty because of the research opportunities that made it so viable. Success followed success in the development of new knowledge which reduced the mortality due to or associated with anesthesia and duly produced the improvement that comes with the influence of outstanding research on the education of people. More and more with each passing year medical and graduate students in the United States and in some Western European countries became increasingly interested in anesthesiology. Major meetings supported by foundations also helped attract people to this now burgeoning specialty. One example was a very important conference sponsored by the Macy Foundation on graduate education in anesthesiology. The leaders of the field were brought together and although there were differences of opinion and not all of the sponsors' staff were totally satisfied with the sharper definition of the need for education, it nonetheless was a great success. Following these discussions there was an interesting unresolved speculation about the elements attractive to young physicians that permitted the American Society of Anesthesiologists to grow by a factor of at least ten fold. The number of Board Diplomates in anesthesiology increased dramatically. There was an infusion of great strength in the clinical anesthetic care of patients. There is no question that the improvement in education, research capability and the drawing together of faculties in academic institutions of stature and competence equal or superior to any of the other clinical fields were major factors in attracting young people. However, one other less spoken and probably less understood aspect of this growth and development was the equality issue where anesthesiologists were put on the same basis as other clinicians in all the conceivable measurable terms. These included fee structures supported by Medicare and by insurance companies. The anesthesiologist suddenly became an earner of very substantial income as a result of the equal treatment of members of this speciality in comparison with those in other clinical fields. This was one of the elements for which I had lobbied for many years. Anesthesiologists were doctors of medicine. They should have equal status with all physicians regardless of other issues. That accomplishment was a major victory for the status and self esteem of anesthesiologists but like so many other things of this sort it quietly permitted the establishment of incomes in excess their sociological worth. A reaction seemed inevitable to some of us and actually set in on 1992 with the suppression and control of the fees of anesthesiologists to a point where it became unattractive to many American graduates of American medical schools.

The accomplishments just described led to other government services in which I had the privilege of participating. I became a member of the Program Project Grants Study Section in the N.I.H., the Pharmacology Study Section, the Surgery Study

Section and eventually the Council of the National Heart Institute as it was called at that time. Services in other parts of the government included chairing the Committee on Anesthesia of the National Research Council and chairing the Sub-committee on Anesthetic Drugs to advise the Food and Drug Administration on these matters. It was a very heady and exciting time to work for the welfare of anesthesiology and for the good of the nation.

ACUPUNCTURE IN THE PEOPLES REPUBLIC OF CHINA: A CULTURAL EXCHANGE MISSION

During the summer of 1974 I had agreed to Chair a delegation sponsored by the National Academy of Sciences to study acupuncture for anesthesia in the People's Republic of China. This was to be the second of nine projected visits that year on an exchange program that was developed between the United States and the People's Republic of China in order to begin what were destined to become satisfactory diplomatic, economic and other types of relationships between the two countries. We were a group of twelve members of the Committee to study acupuncture in China (one can always tell that it is an important committee when the number is the same as the apostolic group of Jesus of Nazareth). We were people who came from several medical disciplines including neurosurgery, neurology, psychiatry, psychology and anesthesiology. There was one individual who was a Chinese scholar. There was excellent staff provided by the National Academy of Sciences. We were in Washington a few days to be briefed about China and about our activities which were planned to bring back new knowledge of acupuncture to the United States thereby to improve relationships between the two countries.

The briefing in Washington of the projected visit to the People's Republic of China as part of the exchange program between the United States and China was excellent. It was due to a very unusual and interesting request by the Chinese asking us to send a team to study the use of acupuncture for surgical anesthesia. They probably made the assumption that experts could be gathered in this country who knew basic things about acupuncture but not its current application to surgical anesthesia. Whatever the underlying reasons of the Chinese were, their part in the mission was entrusted to the Chinese Medical Association, which was to be the host of our delegation. We were told in briefing sessions in Washington that Chairman Mao himself suggested the use of ancient Chinese acupuncture to reinforce Western methods of anesthesia and to marry, as it were, the two cultures from East and West for the benefit of patients. He was also said to have suggested the use of electrical power through the acupuncture needles rather than the simple and ancient custom of twirling the needle in the appropriate meridian. With these thoughts as background it is necessary only to add one other important point which turned out to be a serious factor in our work. The time chosen in 1974 happened to be at the height of the Cultural Revolution in China in which a sort of ethnic cleansing approach was applied not on the basis of ethnicity but on the basis of adherence to the purity of Communist doctrine. We were told to expect a rather harsh repression should there be dissidents among the Chinese professionals with whom we were to work. This prediction was fulfilled more than occasionally during the period of our visit .

As a practical measure to make sense of the observations we were charged with carrying out, our Committee had a balanced presence of different disciplines. I was the Chairperson, or as the Chinese referred to me since titles were abhorrent at the time, the Responsible Person. In some ways their designation was a more powerful and binding one since responsibility carries with it a more awesome burden than being designated a Chairman or Moderator. Our colleagues from the various disciplines were all well known and highly respected scientists or clinicians. To an anesthesiology audience it is of interest to point out that in addition to me there were three other anesthesiologists in the delegation. There were Drs. Francis Foldes, E.S. Siker and Jerome Modell. We all knew each other very well and were good friends. All of which added to the likelihood of our performing a successful mission.

In our planning process, we decided to meet every day prior to an assignment at a hospital or clinic and to meet again after it as soon as possible to discuss our impressions so as to have a fresh view of what we had seen and be able to analyze it more accurately. Some of us — probably most of us — were concerned with deception on the part of our hosts because we came with a preconceived attitude that providing effective surgical anesthesia by American standards was highly unlikely with the use of acupuncture with or without electrical power through the needles. This preconception was to some degree a handicap since it might unfairly influence or bias our deliberations. We thought, probably reasonably, that frequemt open and frank discussions would minimize the likelihood of bias since all of us were strong minded individuals and were totally willing to speak up as to the meanings of our observations. However we took the precaution of having one of us constantly "on duty" to be sure that medicines, drugs or analgesic substances weren't used on the patients without our being informed of it. This aspect of due diligence was a sensible precaution and an important one for us. There was also the serious question raised by some of us about the possibility of a form of self hypnosis or an exaggerated placebo effect because of the strong desire of the relatively simple persons who were patients in the experiments that we were to witness to be "successful" on behalf of Chinese Communism. The essential point of this concern was that a very strong patriotic conviction, either spontaneous or rigidly enforced from the outside, could persuade such patients to put up stoically with pain should it occur during surgical procedures and thereby improve the record of anesthetic power of acupuncture under operating conditions. We understood soon enough why there was this interest on the part of the Chinese, their knowledge at that time and their education, to say nothing of their drugs and equipment, were grossly inferior to the anesthetic capability in North America and in Europe.

With all of these precautions and attitudinal aspects taken into account we began our work in Beijing. We visited important institutions in the nation's capital and were very warmly greeted. The usual custom was for us to gather after breakfast in a conference room around a long table of a type very often pictured in newspapers and in television. The Chinese hosts sat on one side of the longish table and the American visitors on the opposite side. There were soft drinks, tea and many cigarettes lying around, since cigarette smoking was a highly approved practice because Chairman Mao himself was an enthusiastic smoker. Usually what happened was a relatively long speech in three languages before we were to do our practical observations. The first language, at that time called the Common Language and now known by its traditional name, was Mandarin. The second, a recapitulation of the same information was made in the local language (very important for the Chinese since there were so many different languages and dialects in the country and not all of the people were able to understand Mandarin). For our benefit the third summary of all that we were to see and do was then given in English. This practice was repeated at every place we went and, in typical American fashion, we began to put labels on our experiences. The triple header of language became known to us as "the sermon" and to me and two or three others the table packed with American cigarettes was a version of seduction alley. For me this arrangement proved irresistible since I became re-addicted to smoking during that visit to China and was unable to shake the habit until some three years after our return to the United States. The reason for smoking was not only its availability. It was a boring experience when day after day we were given the triple sermon before we could do anything. There was a limit to how much tea one can drink, especially in cool weather when urinary excretion becomes a problem, since it was considered grossly impolite to leave the conference table during the giving of the sermons.

This experience occurred in the many cities and many places we visited. The area was as large as the part of the United States that extends from the Atlantic Ocean to the Mississippi River. We worked very hard for some six weeks and we had many conferences, some of them fiery and some of them rather quiet but all of them truthful and friendly. Despite the fact that all of us saw the same things and heard the same speeches and lectures and talked with the same people, we did not agree on the meaning of our visual and auditory experiences. The majority of us felt that there was a contribution by acupuncture to the production of a state resembling anesthesia but that it did not meet the criteria for useful and practical anesthesia in that one hundred percent satisfactory analgesia, amnesia and patient comfort was achieved in only seventy percent of the procedures that we witnessed. The criterion for satisfactory performance was that there was no addition of any other medication except for local anesthetic infiltration of skin and very superficial tissues. Obviously a seventy percent success record is impressive considering our preconceptions but it is by no means satisfactory by Western standards for surgical anesthesia. We could agree as a group upon that issue.

In searching for mechanisms, we discussed possibilities with our Chinese colleagues in experimental science as well as in clinical medicine. It was suggested by some that an analgesic substance was liberated by the process of acupuncture and discharged into the blood stream. It produced a hormone like substance which had anesthetic properties. These thoughts were explored in rabbit experimentation and a protein derived substance which had anesthetic power was said to have been identified and isolated.

There was a wonderful social aspect to all of these experiences. Our Chinese hosts were very generous and very kind to us and had elaborate and wonderful dinners for us at each place that we visited. We were expected to reciprocate and since the United States government either directly or indirectly did not provide funds for social activities, it was up to the Responsible Person to organize the payment for rather expensive dinners that we gave to our Chinese hosts. They were all very good fun however and very much enjoyed by all of us.

In due course our report was submitted to the National Academy of Sciences. One interesting experience was a consequence of the Cultural Revolution. It can be told since it did not breach any security aspects for the United States. At the time of this incident our delegation was received at the home of the American representative to the People's Republic of China who had neither the status of Ambassador nor of Minister. It was in a period of development of diplomatic relationships so that the United States did not have any recognizable status. The very distinguished and able American Diplomat who had been the United States Ambassador to Paris and I believe to Britain and Germany as well, Mr. David Bruce, was our representative in China. He and Mrs. Evangeline Bruce were truly delightful people. We had a very happy and interesting dinner at their home but apparently there was considerable covert listening by Chinese authorities who had "bugged" the Bruce dwelling. Mr. Bruce at some point was sharply critical of the Communist government. We suffered some concern because of their immediate reaction of putting us under temporary house arrest and removing the symbolic military presence of the United States in China i.e. a few Marines. All cooled off after reasonable apologies and explanations all around and we then proceeded with our work and our journey. I must say that it was a rather tense and somewhat scary moment for us because of the visible disappearance of our Chinese opposite numbers from time to time after having uttered some criticism of the regime either politically and even medically.

Many people have asked about transportation in China at that time. What happened was comparatively straightforward. We flew to Hong Kong and went by train from the New Territories as they were called to the city at that time known as Canton. Most of our travel within China was by fitfully scheduled air transport and by train. We took some short boat rides but these were mostly for sight seeing rather than for actual travel. Our exit from China was in the opposite direction over the same route. We had no problems and no incidents. Everything went off on schedule with the exception of air transport. However, all of the other arrangements were perfectly satisfactory to us.

While in China about midway in our trip, I came down with a respiratory ailment with relatively high fever. I had the unusual experience of being treated with antibiotics and acupressure and recovered in a few days. It was an interesting experience to see Western physicians attribute the recovery to antibiotics and our Eastern Chinese hosts thought that the acupressure paved the way to full recovery. I was briefly hospitalized in a Chinese hospital and must say that treatment was extremely polite, not very modern but very friendly and very comfortable. I view this experience as one the highlights of my own development in education and transcultural affairs!

Toward the end of May of 1974, after my return from China, I plunged back to work in the Dean's office and the resumed difficulties of a widower in Miami. The experience of being the "extra man" at parties, dinners or social occasions was most disagreeable. I had about made up my mind that I would somehow just try to make do with the life that I had as a widower. Then Patricia Meyer Goldstein came into my life.

AUSTRALIA

After deciding to move from the Columbia-Presbyterian Medical Center to the University of Miami School of Medicine as its Dean of the Faculty I thought it would be useful to take a short sabbatical leave of six months to ease the transition for me. While weighing various options a very interesting proposal came to me from the late Professor Douglas Joseph, the Nuffield Professor of anesthesia at the University of Sydney in Australia. He wrote to me suggesting that I should favorably consider coming to Sydney to work as a Visiting Professor at the University of Sydney. I would be assigned to the Royal Prince Alfred Hospital, a major teaching hospital of the University. The visiting professorship had a title as well. It was named in honor of a very distinguished anesthesiologist and a senior person in the Department of Anaesthesiology at the University of Sydney, Dr. Philip Jobson. Before deciding on whether to accept this program I had to get approval first for a sabbatical leave from Dean Merritt at Columbia's College of Physicians and Surgeons as well as the concurrence of Mr. Alvin Binkert who had succeeded John Parke as Executive Vice-President of the Presbyterian Hospital and its Chief Executive Officer. The reason for the need for approval was the fact that the normal sabbatical leave clearly implied a return to the institution and I had planned to use this as a transit period between New York and Miami. Also I had taken only one sabbatical leave in the previous twenty years and that was to work in Washington as the Principal Consultant to Dr. Fred Stone at the National Institute of General Medical Sciences as described elsewhere in this book.

The authorities at the Columbia-Presbyterian Medical Center were very helpful and cooperative and agreed that I could have a sabbatical leave of some six months to work at the University of Sydney and the Royal Prince Alfred Hospital with the clear understanding that I was not returning to the Medical Center in New York.

Professor Joseph suggested that I live in a very large apartment at no cost to me in the Royal Prince Alfred Hospital. He suggested that I should do research work, clinical teaching and provide lectures not only at the University of Sydney but also in other parts of Australia. He was told that other institutions were very anxious to have the first Jobson Professor made available to them. Australians are wonderfully kind and lovable people so that all these plans were going to be accomplished in the most pleasant way. One of the junior members of the department was assigned to me as a sort of aide. We worked together. We shopped together, traveled together and he was of invaluable help to me in many ways. Dr. Colin Shanks is a native of New Zealand who emigrated to Australia and then to the United States.

My work in Australia was very agreeable and while most of it was in Sydney I did have the opportunity of visiting many other parts of that wonderful country and getting to know anesthesiologists in those areas. My lectures, I thought, were kindly and generously well received. My clinical work with the young people of the Sydney Department and the Royal Prince Alfred Hospital staff was very gratifying to me and I think useful to them. My research work was directed at a final opportunity to study renal function in patients in Australia who were anesthetized and operated upon. The population in Australia was an unusual one in that some Australians suffered extensive irreversible damage to the kidneys apparently as a habit of taking large doses of non-opiate analgesic substances for a variety of painful states. The overdose for a long period of time caused so much damage that there were patients with little or no renal function upon whom these studies could be made. The anesthetic effect of drugs upon people with these non functional kidneys was serious. If drug disposition and excretion by the body was dependent upon renal integrity, serious overdose of anesthesia and its consequential damages occurred if great care was not taken to keep these disabilities in mind.

After a very pleasant six months stay in this environment (Julia was with me only part of the time and went to Miami before my return to settle us in so I could get to work as quickly as possible), I returned to Miami just before Christmas of 1969 to take up my duties as Dean of the Faculty of the School of Medicine in that institution. However before I left Australia, my colleagues and friends in Australia were very generous and were most appreciative of my modest efforts on their behalf. We had a succession of dinners to note my stay in Australia and my projected return to the United States. They were kind enough to make me the first Honorary Consultant of the Royal Prince Alfred Hospital since the end of World War II when the Johns Hopkins staff served as clinicians and faculty at that distinguished institution as part of the war effort against Japan. The Australians were very grateful to them and, as is well known, the support of the United States for Australia had changed the orientation of many Australians from Great Britain to the United States.

I also developed a close friendship years later with the distinguished Australian composer, Mr. Peter Sculthorpe, whom I had commissioned while we were both in Aspen, Colorado to write a composition in honor of one of Pat's important birthdays. During the Australian World Congress of 1996 meeting, Peter's composition Kakadu was played together with some of his other work by the Sydney Symphony Orchestra at the beautiful Opera House.

At the meeting of the World Federation of Societies of Anesthesiologists scheduled for April of 1996 in Sydney, the Australian Anaesthesia community very kindly elected me to Fellowship in their Faculty in the Australian and New Zealand College of Anaesthetists.

LIFE AFTER THE COLUMBIA-PRESBYTERIAN MEDICAL CENTER
BECOMING THE DEAN AT THE UNIVERSITY OF MIAMI SCHOOL OF MEDICINE

After some twenty years of serving as Columbia-Presbyterian Medical Center's Chief Executive Officer of the Anesthesiology Program it seemed that my mission was reasonably close to being accomplished and that perhaps I should consider moving to another venue. The student revolutions during the Vietnam War were factors that entered seriously into encouraging my decision to look elsewhere for a new career. I felt singularly upset and alarmed at the student revolutions against the Vietnam War. This was not because I was in favor of the war. Far from it. I served in Vietnam during the height of the violence in 1967 as a "Cinderella General" i.e. as the principal consultant in anesthesiology to the Surgeon-General of the United States Air Force. I saw enough in Vietnam to convince me that the war was immoral, ineffective and would be a major disaster for American military and foreign policy. Things were much worse than the students thought and yet my view was that the major institutions responsible for being repositories of learning should be preserved. If there was protest it should be against the Presi-

dent of the United States, the Congress and the military establishment rather than the civilian guardians of our culture. I felt
that Columbia's President and Board of Trustees were insensi-
tive to better and more effective ways of handling the student
rebellions. If a major institution could be nearly destroyed by a
wrong-headed type of student in upheaval, maybe it was time
for me to move on to one more career that I could enjoy. The
professional reasons for moving, obviously, had to be sound and
reasonable as well.

The question became what to do and when to do it. Fortunately once again in my search for newer opportunities several
were offered. Among them was a very generous suggestion by
William Creasy who was then the Chief Executive Officer of
the Burroughs-Wellcome Company in the United States. At that
time the company was managed by a small committee and a
managing director in London. However, Bill Creasy's American unit earned most of the money granted for research activities and medical aspects of the general welfare. Bill wanted me
to become his vice-president for medical affairs and in charge
of research activities at his splendid company. He was a dear
and close friend and I decided that our friendship was more valuable to me than the possibility that my working for him and for
his company might have led to some strain on that friendship.
He understood and saw my point of view but he also agreed that
I should leave the Columbia-Presbyterian Medical Center for
my own welfare and subsequent "last career" development. There
were several opportunities to chair other departments of anesthesiology which I decided I would not do. There were opportunities in government at the N.I.H. and there were several interesting opportunities to become Dean of a Medical School or the
Chief Executive Officer of an academic hospital. For reasons
that seemed difficult to explain to others I decided that I wanted
to try my skills at the construction of either a new or a very
young school of medicine and its academic health center. This
seemed to be the toughest and yet the most interesting challenge

to face. There were two such opportunities available and I elected to accept the invitation of the University of Miami School of Medicine after about two years of negotiation of matters that were important to me and that I had learned had to be established in advance from my experience at the Columbia-Presbyterian Medical Center in New York. These requirements were finally met. They included the completion of a research building and the moving of the entire school of medicine on to one campus. The School of Medicine was also a very young one having been established and facilitated by the State Legislature in Florida who provided a subsidy to medical students in the school. The subsidy however, was paid to the University of Miami, which made it all financially feasible. It was the first School of Medicine in the state of Florida and yet it was only seventeen years old. It is something of a reflection on how events had changed for me by moving from the oldest established school of Medicine in the United States (even though second to the University of Pennsylvania to confer the M.D. degree) to a very new school that had hardly settled down judging by some of its characteristics. It had separate campuses, the basic science campus at Coral Gables and the clinical campus in downtown Miami. All this was, of course, to be changed. Of much more concern to me were several other facts. In the short existence of the school it had had seventeen deans. To anyone looking at it this was an object of extreme volatility to say nothing of instability. The major teaching hospital of the School of Medicine was a publicly owned county hospital at the time of our negotiations and discussions (and still is). In addition to the problems of management and the difficulties these types of hospitals engender, the physical plant was in very poor condition and needed to be renovated and also considerably strengthened and enlarged to accommodate to practices and clinical care in the 1960s. However on the positive side, the faculty, although small, was distinguished in that its physicians and biomedical scientists were young and vigorously wanted to see the School evolve to a competitive rank among its peers. Also the President of the University, Dr. Henry King Stanford, was an experienced college and university president and was determined to have the School of Medicine flourish and become very good and then excellent. One of its influential trustees, Mr. R. Bunn Gautier, was the State Senator who persuaded the Legislature to provide the funding that I described above and therefore was viewed correctly by all of us as the "father" of the School of Medicine of the University of Miami. Other members of the Board who were close friends with each other and with Mr. Gautier were certainly determined to have their School of Medicine become excellent on the national level and were very generous in their attitudes toward funding from Dade County and from the State of Florida. They had less experience with the federal government but I had had a good deal and we were able to put all our various skills and experience together into a plan of action leading a new School of Medicine to major educational, clinical and reseach strength.

One of the matters that had to be decided as soon as possible was the renovation, expansion and redevelopment of the school's teaching hospital, the Jackson Memorial Hospital, to make its physical development appealing and able to attract more faculty, more students and residents of high quality. This move required a bond issue as the most practical vehicle to secure funding. Dade County decided to embark on what it called "A decade of progress program" that would build this medical center and other cultural and artistic aspects of the county's activities. To secure the funds for the medical center a very large bond issue was planned and was very well documented and described. Many of us, including the then County Manager, Mr. Ray Goode, members of the Board of Trustees, the President, members of our Faculty and I all pitched in together to talk to various clubs lobbying this bond issue. The vote was taken by the public in 1972. The people of Dade County taxed themselves by a two-thirds majority (greater than Nixon's plurality in his second term presidential campaign) to develop a great medical center and other cultural programs, a previously unheard of achievement.

204 – THE PALATE OF MY MIND

One of the great strengths of the young medical school that I had the privilege of leading was its very fine and substantial nucleus of outstanding individuals in several departments. Prominent among these were Bill Whelan, presently a distinguished Fellow of the Royal Society in Britain who was a material force in the research and education of medical and graduate students in biochemistry. In the clinical departments there such stalwarts in medicine as William Harrington, Bob Zeppa in Surgery, Harvey Blank in Dermatology, Ed Norton in Ophthalmology, Peritz Scheinberg in Neurology, Dean Warren in Surgery, Victor Politano in Urology, Gus Sarmiento in Orthopedics and Douglas Anderson in Pathology. It was necessary to support these very able and distinguished individuals to add to their staffs as well as to help them procure and develop laboratory and investigative space on a major scale for an institution that had serious aspirations to national prominence. In due course also there was opportunity to attract very bright, aggressive people (in the best sense of that word) who had a track record of achievement to aid in the development of this young school to a position of excellence.

It was necessary to support financially these new achievements. From a combination of federal, state, county and private sector support the school progressed very rapidly and its people were ready for the new structures which they graced.

It was also highly desirable to strengthen the competence of the student body. The University of Miami, especially its undergraduate body in Coral Gables had an unfortunate and in many ways undeserved reputation as being "Suntan U." The School of Medicine suffered to some extent from this reputation. It was gradually made clear, however, that studying medicine was a serious, time-consuming and difficult occupation. There was no compromise with ability on this issue and gradually and perceptibly a student body of considerable talent was assembled. Their achievements in the various national examinations quickly rose from a lowly to an average performance and eventually to a highly superior one. The upper twenty percent of students could compare favorably with the upper twenty percent in any of the major institutions which with I had experience, including Columbia from whence I came.

The student body's capability was enhanced by a very useful and interesting program designed by Bill Harrington and Bill Whelan to which I lent my energetic support. Individuals who had the Ph.D. degree in fundamental science were able to enter the School of Medicine in modest numbers on a preferred basis. Their time of study was curtailed by approximately twenty five percent by eliminating some of the elective periods which still existed in this School of Medicine. Our expectation was that many of these students would enter academic medicine but the fact is that the number who did fell far below expectation. The program was ended but those of us who had experience with this course look back upon it with satisfaction as a useful experiment and contribution to the school's character and evolution. Many who participated still think it is too bad that the program was not continued.

During much of my period as Dean of the School of Medicine at the University of Miami I was active in securing substantial institutional support from the Florida Legislature in Tallahassee. The trips to the State capital were always interesting and gave me the opportunity and very great pleasure of knowing and forming good friendships with gifted people in the legislature, some of whom became Governor of the State.

On the federal level I had the privilege of enjoying the good friendship of Congressman Paul Rogers who headed the major health related committee in the House of Representatives. We worked very well together and contributed what I think was very valuable substance to the health research of this nation, as well as to the University of Miami School of Medicine. During that phase I was also privileged to have been elected Chairman of the Council of Deans of the American Association of Medical Colleges, the chief organization of academic medicine and to serve as a member of their Executive Council. That position and experience gave me the opportunity of making good friends and learning a great deal from colleagues in all of the Schools of Medicine and the major academic health centers as well as the research institutes of this nation. Most of that knowledge was brought back comfortably and usefully to the School of Medicine at the University of Miami.

Another very important activity of the University of Miami School of Medicine was in international medical education. It was beamed at Latin America and to Spain and Portugal. Miami sits in a strategic position almost athwart North and South America. It also has a very substantial Latin population that has grown to over fifty percent of the Greater Miami area. Most of the Hispanic people in this area are either Cubans or of Cuban descent. However, there is wide representation also of Central and South America as well as a contingent from Spain and a smaller number from Portugal.

President Foote was very much interested in continuing our relationships and our sense of responsibility to our colleagues in Hispanic America and in Europe. His predecessor, Dr. Stanford, also had amply supported our efforts in this direction. By this time a tradition of collaboration and interest in assistance in the medical education of Hispanic America had been formed. It also was an important foreign policy matter for the United States and its obvious medical connections were gratifying both to the North Americans and those who lived in Latin America and in Latin Europe. It was not controversial politically and was therefore very effective.

We had courses which were constructed especially for these constituents of ours. The courses were given in Spanish and in appropriate situations in mixtures of Spanish and English and occasionally there were efforts also to provide for Portuguese speaking people. The language in Brazil and in Portugal did not present any problems because all who were competent physicians were comfortable in either Spanish or in English and usually both. We also had a major effort with medical students from South America in their last student year who joined programs in the Department of Medicine. These were designed to prepare them for internships and possibly residencies at the University of Miami and at other institutions. It was a thriving activity and very successful.

The director of our International Medical Education program was an extraordinary Cuban immigrant, Dr. Rafael Peñalver. He was an experienced internist from Havana and was very bright. [His wonderful personality was ideal for these purposes.] Our personal as well as professional friendship grew rapidly. Because I felt these programs were so important to the School of Medicine I helped him with significant financial as well as intellectual and academic support in every possible way. He always assembled an excellent faculty for the courses in Miami and was very well known and highly regarded in the various institutions we visited together in Latin America. We usually went three times a year to one or more institutions in all parts of Central and South America. We also made one very interesting and important trip to Spain and I also made a trip concerned with Anesthesiology to a joint meeting of the Brazilian and Portuguese Medical Societies.

For these various activities Dr. Peñalver was widely recognized and honored in many of the countries of Central and South America. I was made a Visiting Professor at the Catholic University of Guayaquil in Ecuador and also a distinguished Professor at the University of Madrid in Spain. All these were due to Rafael's influence. One of the very important by products for my own development was a visit that Rafael and I made to the Galapagos Islands off the coast of Ecuador some six hundred miles into the Pacific. This was one of the most fascinating experiences that any person interested in life science could have. Our trip there was in the company of a small number of people and with expert guides. We, in a sense, trod the sacred ground that opened the principles of evolution to Charles Darwin during his epochal voyage on the Beagle.

This program was followed by one in Kuwait where we helped to prepare Kuwaiti physicians for graduate work or residencies in the United States. A Muslim world was a far cry from experiences in Latin America but it was most interesting in a great many ways. Dr. Peñalver's courses adapted into English did succeed in a modest way in achieving the purposes that the Minister of Health in Kuwait wished to accomplish. This was the final effort in our international activities. The program had to be ended after Dr. Peñalver's unfortunately early death from cancer of the colon. His loss to me personally and to the School was very great indeed.

I retired from the Dean's office in 1981 later than I had originally planned to do. President Stanford and I were slated to retire at the same time in 1980 by our own plans and wishes (before it became customary for people to stay on in executive and administrative university positions beyond the age of sixty five). President Foote felt that some bridging was needed and since the medical division was approximately fifty percent of the University of Miami I thought it would be useful to the new President for me to spend another year in helping him get started and delay the selection of the next Dean. [This arrangement turned out to be a happy one for me and a very useful one for President Foote, I believe.] In due course Dr. Bernard Fogel, who had been my assistant, was chosen Dean of the Faculty of Medicine and Senior Vice-President for medical affairs at the University of Miami.

A RETURN TO ANESTHESIOLOGY

After some twelve years of building a powerful medical center, I elected to retire from the position of Dean in 1981. Dr. Brian Craythorne, chairman of the Department of Anesthesiology, was very kind to invite me to participate in several functions. Among them was Chairing the Residency Selection Committee and of behaving in some respects as ombudsman for the resident staff. Pat and I enjoyed having them over to our home for dinner and many things were very pleasant for us in that role. I also had the happy privilege of aiding young members of the Faculty and Attending staff in their work and, finally, of being of use to the departmental Chairman, Dr. Craythorne, in whatever work he asked me to do.

This phase of life is a difficult one for many after being a leader. I found it quite comfortable and easy tbecause the key to happiness is to have one's mind engaged and to be busy and also to of "use." The utilitarian aspect of post power positions is an extraordinarily interesting one and needs to be understood by many people who retain their mental, emotional, and physical agility and other abilities but who no longer have power. It is much more interesting in many respects to be of use and have influence than to have power.

The experience of working with young people once again in a close and intimate fashion was a very important and stimulating one for me and I think a useful one for them, because in one of those interesting years they chose me as their as outstanding teacher of the year! It was not always the substance that one transferred to young people or guided them to achieving but it was the feeling of friendship and warmth with them that gave them the impression, I was about to say illusion, of having been taught something. Maybe they learned a great deal that was important. They said so. I think I stimulated them to want to learn and that is probably a more successful experience from an educational standpoint than the standard way of teaching residents.

I began to go to anesthesiology meetings again and had the very great pleasure of renewing old friendships both here and abroad as well as becoming friendly with some of the bright new people in many institutions. I resumed attending international meetings in anesthesiology as well and enjoyed very much the companionship of very dear and wonderful friends in many parts of the world. My strong mental engagement with the newer aspects of anesthesiology, with fundamental science and with the improvement of clinical care gave me great pleasure. I also began to long to return to the discipline in the Humanities that I had thought was going to be my life experience and which started at Columbia College some fifty years earlier. I spent a considerable amount of time as a participant in various seminars in the

Aspen Institute for Humanistic Studies and renewed many of my friendships with people like Mortimer Adler, to whom I became very devoted. The friendship was mutual. I began to focus a bit more on certain aspects of the beginnings of anesthesia as a therapeutic weapon.

I had always been unimpressed by the historical version of how the most unlikely people were the principal actors in the drama of the "discovery" of anesthesia. However, I had to change my agreeable dilettante reading habits to focus on this issue.

It became increasingly obvious that my reading in various aspects of the humanities was undirected and, although very pleasant, wasn't focused. In order to sharpen the direction of my reading, I thought it would be of interest to explore why the discovery of anesthesia happened so peculiarly late in Western civilization. Fom a humanitarian point of view I made the obvious and clear assumption that all people would have very much wanted to find a way of preventing the awful, searing pain of surgical operation. I assumed that everyone preferred to have maximum comfort for patients. I also was aware that it might be a difficult problem since scientific medicine, as we know it, is a relatively recent addition to our culture. Scientific medicine really begins only with the development of microscopic pathology and microbiology which made it possible to find specific causes for certain illnesses.

As I began to do serious reading in the basic question of why it took so long to develop pain prevention methods against surgical operation, I began to realize that I had to seek further knowledge away from the polemics of who discovered anesthesia and try to understand some of its cultural relationships. The assumption that everyone wanted to prevent the pain of surgery had to be examined. The furor over the priority of "the discovery" was not going to enlighten me about my question of why it took so long.

My concerns were further deepened by the puzzling fact that anesthetic agents had been known for a very long time and yet nothing practical had come of these discoveries. For instance, ether was well known as early as 1540, discovered by a young Prussian scientist known as Valerius Cordus. Nitrous oxide had been developed by Joseph Priestly in 1772 and also had never been used for anesthesia even though the famous chemist Sir Humphry Davy experimented with it at the age of nineteen while working in the famous Pneumatic Institute created and managed by Dr. Thomas Beddoes Sr. It finally occurred to me that the assumption that there was a prolonged search for appropriate anesthetic drugs so that the humanitarian instincts of western society could be satisfied, was erroneous. Those who are interested can explore this subject in a book that I published in 1995, entitled *Romance, Poetry, and Surgical Sleep — Literature Influences Medicine* (Greenwood Publishing Group).

I decided that one of the possible sources of further information would be in literature and certainly other of the arts. My taste of course ran to looking at literature and this posed another problem. What does one read? How do you go about finding your way? There are many answers to this kind of problem but I had another chance opportunity and capitalized on it.

One of my friends invited me to a lunch at which members of the university of Miami's English Department were to be present. By sheer good fortune, among them was a very capable and energetic faculty member, Professor Hermione de Almeida, who eventually functioned as my thesis advisor when I became a graduate student in the Department of English. I also met her husband, Professor George Gilpin and learned from them that I had a good chance of getting the insights I was searching for if I took some course work in the literature of the early nineteenth century in Great Britain and in the United States. However, they cautioned me that it would be difficult to step into a reading of structured literature at that point because to understand the Romantic Period one had to understand the Enlightenment of the eighteenth century. To understand that period one had to know something of medieval literature and so on and so forth. I was therefore advised to become a formal graduate student and a Ph.D. candidate in English Literature. Taking their advice, I set about becoming a graduate student at the age of seventy and found it extraordinarily exciting and stimulating. I met wonderful bright young people who were dedicated to careers in English Literature and who were very friendly and very helpful. Our classes were usually between ten and fifteen students in size and our faculty was very strong and distinguished. This department had six internationally renowned Joyce scholars and one would be silly, even though it wasn't a direct interest of mine, not to take advantage of learning all one could about the very distinguished literary artist, James Joyce. Many of us took all the courses available on Joyce. I also embarked on studies in the classics of Greece and Rome followed by the literature of the Dark Ages and continued into medieval literature and then the Enlightenment of the Eighteenth century. With this background I was able to study the Romantics more intelligently and decided to do my doctoral dissertation on British Romantic poets with whom I found the kinds of insights that I was searching for.

To summarize the story perhaps inadequately, it appeared to me that the subjectivity and the emotional charge of British Romantic literature, especially in its poetry, showed very clearly that care and attention for the individual was a necessity if one wanted to do something useful to prevent pain and suffering. Furthermore, it required a democratic society in which people cared for individuals and wanted to be helpful. For such a society to flourish required clear understanding and possession of certain fundamental rights which grew out of the Enlightenment of the eighteenth century. It is interesting to note that the very first teaching hospital in western society was established in Paris in 1796 as part of the thrust to democracy and belief in equality of the French Revolution. Furthermore, I found no evidence that the ancients in classic Greece or Rome cared very much about the individual. Their attitudes to pain and suffering were cosmic in nature and were closely linked to fate and the decisions of the gods. In the other part of our western traditions, Judaism and Christianity, there was also a clear train of evidence that pain and suffering was meted out by a vengeful God as punishment for sin. This particular aspect of religious inheritance provoked very stern opposition to doing anything about pain relief and prevention because it conflicted with the will of God. Christianity added that to be martyred for Christ was a guarantee of eternal salvation in Heaven, which was obviously a more happy alternative than the miserable life that so many people led on earth in the ages that preceded the Romantic Period.

The Romantic Period, while setting the stage for the development of anesthesia, from a societal point of view, also had its problems. Shortly thereafter the Industrial Revolution came along and many of the gains made in the individual rights of man were blunted by a new form of slavery in the factory workplace.

These concepts are new and certainly controversial. However, I had a wonderful time doing the study. I succeeded in passing the qualifying examinations and ultimately defended a doctoral dissertation on this very subject. The Ph.D. was awarded on my seventy-fifth birthday in 1990.

I had the opportunity through my thesis advisor, Professor de Almeida, to meet experts in the area of criticism of the British Romantics. All in all it was a delightful experience and one that continues to this very day in connection with what I read and what I write. I hope some of it shows in this memoir!

Among my newer literary friends was the distinguished writer whose marvelous book *How we Die* won the National Book Award for 1995, Dr. Sherwin B. Nuland. He had recently retired from the Yale Department of Surgery in New Haven, Connecticut. I also continued to work in a modest way in maintaining my very happy connections with the College of Physicians and Surgeons at Columbia and Columbia College. My additional responsibilities in foundation consultation work were modest in size but very rewarding in result.

We had produced a very good resident staff for the Department at the University of Miami and all of us were happy with the excellent conduct of anesthesia and the experience of edu-

214 - THE PALATE OF MY MIND

cating young bright young people. In 1992 the story changed abruptly and drastically for the worse.

Suddenly, there was a marked fall off in graduates of American medical schools who up to that date had entered the specialty of anesthesiology in substantial numbers.

What we are seeing is apparently a part of the massive revolution in the practice of medicine that occurred beginning in 1992 and is still going on strongly in 1996. In my judgment this in not the time for finger pointing or blame assessment but it should precipitate and produce serious attempts at some analysis of what has happened, what is likely to happen and what remedies can be proposed for rectification of what looks like a massive overcorrection of a problem that needed attention. I refer, of course, to the legitimate concerns about vast escalation of the cost of medical care to a society that is wealthy but does not have unlimited resources. The various attempts at cost containment in the hands of the medical profession apparently were ineffective as were the attempts to provide sensible medical care to all Americans without adding to the cost while preserving the quality. The entire country seemed to be suddenly engulfed by a tidal wave of private sector participation in the ownership of for-profit hospitals as well as the introduction of large numbers of HMO establishments controlled by managed care methods also in the private sector.

I do not know whether studies have been complete enough or sharp enough to indicate if things truly are troublesome but it seems pretty clear that major cost containment has not occurred and that the quality of medical care has declined. There is clear evidence of disruption of an important part of medical care, the relationship between physician and patient, which seems to be in a state of chaos.

Anesthesiology as a specialty has perhaps been hardest hit among all those affected by these changes of the medical revolution in which we are engaged. The main streams of the problem for anesthesiology seem to be an over supply of anesthesiologists and a position of real captivity in the economic sense where anesthesiologists either singly or in groups can be aggressively pushed by the managed care structures to which they are subject. I find it hard to believe that there is an oversupply of anesthesiologists if one is able to accept my basic thesis that for anesthetic care every patient deserves a well trained *physician* who is a specialist in anesthesiology. I know that this will once again produce storms of protest about nurse anesthetists. I may have to modify my point of view about oversupply because that deals necessarily with a conflict between ideal, as I view it, and reality as it presently exists in this country. The issue of a victim group captive of managed care economics is a real one and I doubt that anyone could dispute that fact.

What to do about it is subject to considerable discussion and will be for a long time to come. I find it a very saddening experience in at least two important respects. One of them is personal. Despite a life given over to advancing anesthesiology — and, it seemed, very productively — I am now in the position where I wonder whether all of my time, effort and work has come to naught. Our specialty is essentially beaten into ineffectiveness by these economic forces. There are those who would maintain that we are the victims of our own success. Reducing mortality so sharply from an estimated one in six thousand anesthetics delivered to approximately one in four hundred thousand is breath taking in its implications. This achievement is more dramatic than what we have done in the control of poliomyelitis and tuberculosis and certainly is more spectacular than what we have achieved so far in the control of AIDS. And yet despite these magnificent achievements here is a group of doctors destined for the fate of dinosaurs unless something is done to preserve the progress that has been made and to extend it further. Research needs to go on. Clinical care still needs to be improved and education still needs greater support. How all this will be done in the present environment is difficult to imagine. I live in the expectation that this marked overcorrection, which resulted in part from the greed of anesthesiologists in private and academic practice, will one day settle into a middle path for the benefit of the anesthetic care of our nation. This process could take a few years or many years but I do believe that it is inevitable. Anesthesiologists are needed. They must not suffer the fate of dinosaurs.

EPILOGUE

As the writing of this memoir neared its end, I began to think much more often than previously of how to interpret my fifty six years in anesthesiology. The career from its beginnings until the early 1990's participatied in the development of anesthesiology to a level of excellence and great accomplishment for the public welfare. This process saw compassion for patients retained and high technology introduced to monitor and treat events as they arose during the course of clinical anesthesia in patients. I felt particularly fortunate in the middle years of this period at being of some importance in helping to organize a major research effort in anesthesiology that was a momentous source of clinical care of patients. It helped to sharply lower the mortality due to anesthesia. and enabled the opening of many new areas of operative surgery, intensive care, and pain management. Entire fields of surgery never before performed were made possible by a combination of fundamental research in each of the surgical and medically related fields as well as the crucial role of anesthesia. Excellent anesthesia enabled patients to survive in good condition after increasingly difficult surgical procedures, transplantation of organs including the heart, and bold surgical interventions in people previously deemed too ill for such care.

How to think about the dramatically changing events is very difficult. I have a natural revulsion for the possibility that this field will no longer exist. My belief, however, is that in the face of obstacles the need for excellent anesthesia will be, once again, appreciated as crucial for society.

My expectation is that a democratic society will eventually find a middle ground. In the worst possible case the accomplishments of anesthesiology and my participation, which gave me very great pleasure, have been major enough to be an immortal part of American and world medicine. In the best possible case there is still much room to evolve towards improvement in patient care with the aid of scientific research. A society cannot be forever so blunted against its own self interest as to permit what we are seeing today to endure.